Veterinary Clinical Skills

Veterinary Clinical Skills

Edited by

Emma K. Read, DVM, MVSc, DACVS
College of Veterinary Medicine, The Ohio State University
Columbus, OH, USA

Matt R. Read, DVM, MVSc, DACVAA
MedVet, Worthington, OH, USA

Sarah Baillie, BVSc, PhD, MRCVS
Bristol Veterinary School, University of Bristol
Bristol, UK

WILEY Blackwell

Registered Office
John Wiley & Sons, Inc., 111 River Street, Hoboken, NJ 07030, USA

Editorial Office
111 River Street, Hoboken, NJ 07030, USA

For details of our global editorial offices, customer services, and more information about Wiley products visit us at www.wiley.com.

Wiley also publishes its books in a variety of electronic formats and by print-on-demand. Some content that appears in standard print versions of this book may not be available in other formats.

Library of Congress Cataloging-in-Publication Data

Names: Read, Emma K., editor. | Read, Matt R., editor. | Baillie, Sarah, editor.
Title: Veterinary clinical skills / edited by Emma K. Read, Matt R. Read, Sarah Baillie.
Description: First edition. | Hoboken, NJ : John Wiley & Sons, Inc., 2022.
Identifiers: LCCN 2021032454 (print) | LCCN 2021032455 (ebook) | ISBN 9781119540052 (paperback) | ISBN 9781119540144 (adobe pdf) | ISBN 9781119540151 (epub)
Subjects: MESH: Education, Veterinary | Clinical Competence
Classification: LCC SF756.3 (print) | LCC SF756.3 (ebook) | NLM SF 756.3 | DDC 636.089/0711–dc23
LC record available at https://lccn.loc.gov/2021032454
LC ebook record available at https://lccn.loc.gov/2021032455

Cover Design: Wiley
Cover Images: © Emma K. Read, Matt R. Read

Set in 9.5/12.5pt STIXTwoText by Straive, Pondicherry, India

Contents

Acknowledgments

This work would not have been possible without the contributions of many colleagues with whom we have worked over the years. We are grateful to the efforts of so many talented instructors and staff members in making our clinical skills training programs a reality. We are also delighted to have had the opportunity to watch our learners grow and mature into competent and caring practitioners. Thank you to them for taking care of the profession, animals, and their owners on a daily basis. Your work is difficult and vitally important.

We would also like to recognize the team at Wiley, specifically Erica Judisch and Merryl Le Roux. We have enjoyed working with you and appreciate your tremendous support on this project since from the beginning.

Emma

Thanks to my parents and family members who always supported me and helped me to achieve my career aspirations by encouraging me to work hard and seek out broad opportunities to learn. Thanks to my husband Matt for his unfailing support of all my projects and dreams, and for being my rock along the way.

To our co-editor, Sarah, a special thanks for being such a wonderful collaborator and friend over the years. We feel very fortunate to have met you and have really enjoyed working with you ever since.

To Grace and Kate, thank you above all else. You are the light of our lives. Words can't express the love we have for you or our admiration for the people you are. Your patience with our many work hours, projects, and life changes are so appreciated. We love you with all our hearts. Chase your dreams with all your being – we are here for you!

Matt

For my incredible wife, Emma, for having the vision and passion to create this book despite everything else going on around us. I learn something new from you every single day. But enough with the summative assessments already!

For our two daughters, Grace and Kate. I am looking forward to again using evenings and weekends for the things you want to do! You are simply amazing and I am so thankful to be your dad.

And to my parents and friends who have supported and helped me through thick and thin. Life can be hard, but you make it easier.

Sarah

Thanks to Emma for inviting me to join this project, it is one of many we have collaborated on over the years. It has been a pleasure as always. Thanks to my husband John who is so supportive in so many ways in all my endeavors at work and at home. And finally this book, and my ongoing enthusiasm for "all things" clinical skills, wouldn't be such fun without all the help from my colleagues in the clinical skills lab team at Bristol.

List of Contributors

Stacy L. Anderson
College of Veterinary Medicine
Lincoln Memorial University
Harrogate, TN, USA

Elizabeth Armitage-Chan
LIVE Centre, Department of Clinical Sciences
and Services
Royal Veterinary College
Hatfield
UK

Sarah Baillie
Bristol Veterinary School
University of Bristol
Bristol, UK

Teresa Burns
College of Veterinary Medicine
The Ohio State University
Columbus, OH
USA

Alison Catterall
Bristol Veterinary School
University of Bristol
Bristol
UK

Kate Cobb
School of Veterinary Medicine and Science
University of Nottingham
Sutton Bonington
UK

Sarah Cripps
School of Veterinary Medicine and Science
University of Nottingham
Sutton Bonington
UK

Marc Dilly
Faculty of Veterinary Medicine
Justus Liebig University Giessen
Giessen
Germany

Robin Farrell
UCD School of Veterinary Medicine
University College Dublin
Dublin
Ireland

Andrew Gardiner
Royal (Dick) School of Veterinary Studies
University of Edinburgh
Scotland
UK

Rachel Harris
Bristol Veterinary School
University of Bristol
Bristol
UK

Jennifer Hodgson
Virginia-Maryland College of Veterinary
Medicine
Virginia Tech
Blacksburg, VA
USA

Steven Horvath
College of Veterinary Medicine
The Ohio State University
Columbus, OH
USA

Julie A. Hunt
College of Veterinary Medicine
Lincoln Memorial University
Harrogate, TN
USA

Keshia John
School of Veterinary Medicine
St. George's University
Grenada
West Indies

Jennifer T. Johnson
College of Veterinary Medicine
Lincoln Memorial University
Harrogate, TN
USA

Rikke Langebæk
Department of Veterinary Clinical Science
University of Copenhagen
Copenhagen
Denmark

Rachel Lumbis
Royal Veterinary College
Hatfield
UK

Susan M. Matthew
Department of Veterinary Clinical Sciences,
College of Veterinary Medicine
Washington State University
Pullman, WA
USA

Missy Matusicky
College of Veterinary Medicine
The Ohio State University
Columbus, OH
USA

Catherine May
Faculty of Veterinary Science
University of Pretoria
Pretoria, South Africa

Tatiana Motta
College of Veterinary Medicine
The Ohio State University
Columbus, OH
USA

Máire O'Reilly
University College Dublin
Dublin
Ireland

Carolina Ricco Pereira
College of Veterinary Medicine
The Ohio State University
Columbus, OH
USA

Megan Preston
College of Veterinary Medicine
Lincoln Memorial University
Harrogate, TN
USA

Lindsey Ramirez
College of Veterinary Medicine
Lincoln Memorial University
Harrogate, TN
USA

Emma K. Read
College of Veterinary Medicine
The Ohio State University
Columbus, OH
USA

Matt R. Read
MedVet
Worthington, OH
USA

Alfredo E. Romero
Faculty of Veterinary Medicine
University of Calgary
Calgary, Alberta
Canada

Elrien Scheepers
Faculty of Veterinary Science
University of Pretoria
Pretoria, RSA

Jennifer Schleining
College of Veterinary Medicine & Biomedical
Sciences
Texas A&M University
College Station, TX
USA

Lucy Squire
Bristol Veterinary School,
University of Bristol
Bristol
UK

Jean-Yin Tan
Faculty of Veterinary Medicine
University of Calgary
Calgary, Alberta
Canada

Abi Taylor
College of Veterinary Medicine
North Carolina State University
Raleigh, NC
USA

Sheena Warman
Bristol Veterinary School,
University of Bristol
Bristol
UK

Catherine Werners
School of Veterinary Medicine
St. George's University
Grenada
West Indies

Lissann Wolfe
School of Veterinary Medicine
College of Medical, Veterinary & Life Sciences
University of Glasgow
Glasgow
UK

Preface

Our original vision for this book was to try to collate the content of many years of conversations that we have had with colleagues and students about Clinical Skills teaching and learning into a single, useful resource. Many of those discussions centered around what is known about how to teach and learn better – in essence, where to spend one's precious time, effort, and resources in order to see the best returns. To this end, we wanted to create a book that would appeal to both instructors and students and provide a broad overview of what is already known about teaching and learning Clinical Skills for those starting out so they had a good base from which to take the leap.

We have been fortunate to help institute modern clinical skills training programs into our own institutions at a time when they were just beginning to be implemented across veterinary medicine. In the early days, we learned by trial and error by adapting "hard knocks" lessons we had learned in private practice to our academic learning environments. As programs evolved, so did the research that proves that there is value in learning how to use best teaching practices to inform Clinical Skills instruction. However, even though so much has been published, clinical skills instructors are a generous group and much of the sharing of information still tends to be open source or available by simply asking a colleague. Websites, conferences, and Zoom calls all serve as a means for sharing what we have learned, making sure that someone else does not have to reinvent the wheel.

The basis for this book is that, despite all of the sharing of ideas and best practices that has occurred to date (or maybe as a result of it!), it can still be challenging for instructors and students to review what has been documented about teaching and learning Clinical Skills in one concise place. New instructors often feel overwhelmed with all there is to know about teaching and assessment and, although many teachers may not be new to veterinary medicine or to teaching Clinical Skills, it is the evidence-based teaching of others that is novel and challenging. Students tackling clinical skills training are often overwhelmed with where to begin and how best to practice the huge volume of skills and procedures that a veterinarian needs to be able to perform following graduation. Although handbooks have been published that list skills and explain "how to" perform a variety of procedures, a concise reference that summarizes all that is known about teaching, learning, and assessing clinical skills all in one place has still been missing.

We hope that this book helps point newbies of all types in the right direction while also serving as a go-to reference for experienced teachers. The enthusiasm and dedication to clinical skills training is as evident now as it was when it started over 10 years ago and we are immensely grateful to all of the authors who participated in this project and shared their expertise and experiences so openly. Together, we look forward to further innovations that will make even more confident and competent day-one graduates who will be better prepared to treat the animals in their care.

About the Companion Website

This book is accompanied by a companion website:

www.wiley.com/go/read/veterinary

There you will find valuable material designed to enhance your learning, including:

- Appendices 1 and 2 from the book as downloadable PDF

1

What Is a Clinical Skill?

Emma K. Read[1] and Sarah Baillie[2]

[1] College of Veterinary Medicine, The Ohio State University, Columbus, OH, USA
[2] Bristol Veterinary School, University of Bristol, Bristol, UK

Historically in veterinary medicine, degree programs have been based upon the Flexner model described in medical education, with two basic blocks: two to three years of preclinical training and one to two years of clinical training (Flexner, 1910). Approximately 10–15 years ago, a trend developed in veterinary education to include more hands-on training during veterinary programs, often beginning in the start of the first year, with an emphasis on teaching day-one skills necessary for success in practice (Hubbell et al., 2008; Doucet and Vrins, 2009; Welsh et al., 2009; Smeak et al., 2012; Dilly et al., 2017 RCVS, 2020;). The idea of moving clinical training earlier in the program and further emphasizing integration of knowledge and other skills into the clinical workplace led to current veterinary programs being more like two inverse wedges rather than two blocks placed one on top of the other as separate units of the same program (Figure 1.1).

Formal veterinary clinical skills training programs, which emphasized the use of models and simulators and constructed dedicated clinical skills centers for teaching, began in the early to mid-2000s as a way to accommodate this need for earlier training (Baillie et al., 2005; Scalese and Issenberg, 2005; Pirkelbauer et al., 2008; Read and Hecker, 2013; Dilly et al., 2017). Reports of objective structured clinical examinations (OSCEs) that are used to assess learners' hands-on skills, and descriptions of best practices for implementing skills curricula, began to follow (Smeak, 2007; Rhind et al., 2008; May and Head, 2010; Hecker et al., 2010; Read and Hecker, 2013; Dilly et al., 2017).

Concurrently, over the last 10 years, there has been a recognition of the need to incorporate more professional skills training (NAVMEC, 2011; Cake et al., 2016). Today's employers are not only searching for confidence and technical competence in new graduates but good communication abilities as well (Perrin, 2019). Rather than simply being competent in one's hands-on skills alone, effective integration of professional communication and technical skills performance is crucial for successful practice (NAVMEC, 2011; Rhind et al., 2011). Other "marketable skills" described in a recent report of the characteristics most often sought by employers posting job advertisements in the United Kingdom included enthusiasm, special interest, communication, all-rounder, client care, team player, autonomous, caring, ambitious, and high clinical standards (Perrin, 2019). These "skills" are important to employers and are key to minimizing dissonance and dissatisfaction for the graduates as well (May, 2015; Perrin, 2019).

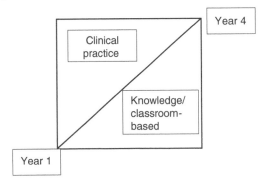

Figure 1.1 Flexner model (with separation between preclinical and clinical blocks) versus the more recent curricular models that are more like inverse wedges introducing clinical content earlier into the start of the curriculum.

The Royal College of Veterinary Surgeons (RCVS) Day One Competences and the American Association of Veterinary Medical Colleges' (AAVMC) North American Veterinary Medical Education Consortium (NAVMEC) report are both recognized as early frameworks that defined competencies across a number of areas that lead to graduate success (NAVMEC, 2011 RCVS, 2020;). More recently, there have been other developments toward employability of new graduates and improved teaching of professional skills. The VetSet2Go project represents an international collaboration of educators (https://www.vetset2go.edu.au), who surveyed employers, clients, new graduates, and other stakeholders before combining this information with what was already published in the literature. The resulting white paper and framework have been used to guide development of resources, as well as tools for educators and learners (Cake et al., 2016; Hughes et al., 2018). This framework highlights professional identity formation, skills needed for practice career longevity, and development of resilience. More recently, outcomes-based frameworks have been described (Bok et al., 2011; Molgaard et al., 2019; Matthew et al., 2020). The AAVMC's competency-based veterinary education (CBVE) framework is currently being considered and implemented across multiple international veterinary schools simultaneously, which brings exciting opportu-

nities for conducting comparative analysis of students and graduates across schools. Having a shared framework of competencies, entrustable professional activities, milestones, and terminology is critical for training educators, comparing learners, and generalizing results across programs (Molgaard et al., 2018a; Molgaard et al., 2018b; Salisbury et al., 2019). With schools historically only focusing on their own programs, this opportunity has not existed in veterinary medicine to date.

In the strictest sense, veterinary clinical skills are psychomotor tasks that can be assessed in a simulated environment (satisfying "shows how" on Miller's pyramid of clinical competence) or within the actual clinical workplace (satisfying "does" on Miller's pyramid of clinical competence, see Figure 5.1) (Miller, 1990). Obvious examples might include donning and doffing a surgical gown, suturing skin, performing venipuncture, safely restraining a patient, or performing a complete physical examination. But what about interpreting herd records, observing animal behavior, or designing an isolation facility? Recently, authors have argued that the pinnacle of Miller's pyramid of clinical competence is not just related to technical skill competence as Miller originally described but is actually "is trusted" (to perform on one's own) (ten Cate et al., 2020) or "is" (to incorporate the development of professional identity) (Cruess et al., 2016).

During curriculum development or program revision to incorporate further clinical skills training, there can be heated debate among educators and practitioners about what skills are the most necessary to teach, or even about what constitutes a "clinical skill." Before the more recent rise of competency-based education, some educators and practitioners used Delphi-like processes and developed lists of skills to be taught in veterinary programs such as Day 1 Skills, first published in 2002 (RCVS, 2020). These practitioners tended to focus on what they believed was important for their own daily practice and based the skills list on what might be needed for their particular geographical location. Practitioners also focused on what they wished to be taught to students who were soon to become their employees and colleagues. Educators tended to focus more on their own areas of specialty and what they believed new graduates should be able to perform based on past teaching experience.

The more recently described competency-based approaches to education have tried to focus more on "outputs," rather than only on "inputs" for determining what should be taught in the curriculum. The majority of veterinary graduates today will enter private small animal, first-opinion practice, and it has been suggested that educators focus on asking practitioners working in that environment what skills the graduate will need (Bain and Salois, 2019). It should be noted that a broad range of practices must be consulted because there are differences in equipment and personnel available from practice to practice. Surveys of practicing veterinarians engaged in performing authentic veterinary tasks in general practice have also proven critical to determining the frequency, importance, and perceived difficulty for performance of these skills (Hubbell et al., 2008; Doucet and Vrins, 2009; Smeak et al., 2012; Luby et al., 2013; Kreisler et al., 2019). Not being limited in licensure at present, veterinary graduates ultimately require a broad range of skills for commonly seen conditions and diseases of all the major domestic species, and they require different skills than a specialist working in a tertiary referral environment (May, 2015). It is critically important that information be gathered across all types of practice, and published surveys exist in the literature for skills in surgery, equine practice, bovine practice, and small animal practice (Hubbell et al., 2008; Doucet and Vrins, 2009; Smeak et al., 2012; Luby et al., 2013; Kreisler et al., 2019). These resources are very useful and essential to consult when considering what to incorporate into an educational program.

Integration of clinical skills in the curriculum requires consideration of when to present the material and whether to integrate it with other competencies. It is not enough for learners to learn the technical performance alone because without the knowledge of when to use the skill, when not to use the skill and how to modify the performance of the skill when needed, then the learner performs as a trained technician (Michels et al., 2012). The development of a veterinary professional requires that the learner has declarative or background knowledge, procedural knowledge about how to perform the skill, and can also apply diagnostic reasoning and clinical decision-making. In effect, developing a clinical skills program means achieving a comprehensive consensus on all of these aspects and not simply generating a list of skills (Michels et al., 2012).

Initially, the emphasis of outcomes-based education in the health professions was on the postgraduate learner, but more recently there has been a shift to incorporate undergraduate training as well (Ferguson et al., 2017). The competency-based educational approach supports the continual documented improvement of learner performance from novice to proficient and emphasizes training in the clinical workplace (Dreyfus, 2004). Assessment is becoming increasingly focused on a programmatic approach that includes multiple direct observations of student performance that are then integrated to provide a complete picture of learner competence (Bok et al., 2018; Norcini et al., 2018; van Melle et al., 2019).

The development of entrustable professional activities (EPAs) is ushering in a new era for skills training where students are ultimately encouraged to bring individual skills and competencies together in a comprehensive authentic workplace procedural performance (ten Cate, 2005). EPAs are activities that are performed in the workplace and offer a chance for observation and assessment. Assessors have a chance to observe "in the moment" and comment on the learner's ability to perform tasks required in practice. The repetitious completion of such activities in the clinical veterinary teaching environment allows the trainee to grow and learn from the formative feedback provided to them. The AAVMC's CBVE working group recently defined nine different domains and 32 competencies in a framework, which represents consensus across a number of veterinary programs (Molgaard et al., 2018a; Molgaard et al., 2018b). The group then described eight EPAs that can be used for assessing and documenting learner development during the clinical years of the training program. Clinical skills training is now evaluated across programs through the use of OSCEs to assess introductory individual skills and short procedures in the years prior to clinical rotations, and EPAs and workplace-based assessments that evaluate more complex procedures or activities where multiple competencies need to be performed simultaneously in the clinical environment (Petersa et al., 2017; ten Cate et al., 2018; Molgaard et al., 2018b).

Programmatic assessment has recently been validated in veterinary medicine and shows that a change in performance is not simply due to variability between raters but is due to variance in learners' growth (Bok et al., 2018). This is important because we can now demonstrate learner change over time and predict the rate at which mastery will occur (Pusic et al., 2015). Limitations of accreditation (e.g. American Veterianry Medical Association's Council on Education mandating the maintenance of a four-year program) and reduced financial support (e.g. in the United States, many colleges have poor public support and rely heavily on tuition dollars) may mean that true time-independent advancement may prove challenging for veterinary programs.

In summary, veterinarians used to talk about "see one, do one, teach one," but today this is no longer considered a valid approach to teaching and learning skills (Michels et al., 2012). Clinical skills teaching, learning, and assessment have evolved. There is a growing body of evidence regarding learning theories, teaching and assessment principles, and learner development that can be used to the advantage of learner, teacher, and other stakeholders. An abundance of research and scholarship has changed the way that educators teach and the way programs are designed. This book is intended to focus on teaching, learning, and assessment of clinical skills in the modern veterinary curriculum and is a resource guide for students, as well as their instructors. This book is written for both veterinary and veterinary nursing students and includes chapters regarding development of skills curriculum (Chapter 2), how skills are best taught and learned (Chapter 3), and how skills are best practiced prior to assessment (Chapter 4). Also included are chapters on how learners know if they are learning what they need to (Chapter 5), how learners know they are being assessed fairly (Chapter 6), how learners can best learn in a simulated environment (Chapter 7), how to make use of peer teachers (Chapter 8), and what other skills are vital to a successful practice career (Chapter 9). The appendices include examples of OSCE assessments and recipes for simple models that instructors and learners can use and make.

References

Baillie, S., Crossan, A., Brewster, S., et al. 2005. Validation of a bovine rectal palpation simulator for training veterinary students. *Stud Health Technol Inform*, 111, 33–36.

Bain, B., Salois, M. 2019. Employment, starting salaries, and educational indebtedness of year-2018 graduates of US veterinary medical colleges. *J Am Vet Med Assoc*, 254, 1061–1066.

Bok, H., Jaarsma, D., Tenuissen, P., et al. 2011. Development and validation of a competency framework for veterinarians. *J Vet Med Educ*, 38, 262–269.

Bok, H., de Jong, L., O'Neill, T., et al. 2018. Validity evidence for programmatic assessment in competency-based education. *Perspect Med Educ*, 7, 362–372.

Cake, M., Bell, M., Williams, J., et al. 2016. Which professional (non-technical) competencies are most important to the success of graduate veterinarians? A Best Evidence Medical Education (BEME) systematic review: BEME guide no. 38. *Med Teach*, 38, 550–563.

Cruess, R. L., Cruess, S. R., Steinert, Y. 2016. Amending Millers' pyramid to include professional identity formation. *Acad Med*, 91, 180–185.

Dilly, M., Read, E., Baillie, S. 2017. A survey of established veterinary clinical skills laboratories from Europe and North America: Present practices and recent developments. *J Vet Med Educ*, 44, 580–589.

Doucet, M., Vrins, A. 2009. The importance of knowledge, skills, and attitude attributes for veterinarians in clinical and non-clinical fields of practice: A survey of licensed veterinarians in Quebec, Canada. *J Vet Med Educ*, 36, 331–342.

Dreyfus, S. E. 2004. The five-stage model of adult skill acquisition. *Bull Sci Technol Soc*, 24, 177–181.

Ferguson, P., Caverzagie, K., Nousiainen, M., et al. 2017. Changing the culture of medical training: An important step toward the implementation of competency-based medical education. *Med Teach*, 39, 599–602.

Flexner, A. 1910. Medical education in the United States and Canada. *Bull World Health Org*, 80, 594–602, extracted from Bulletin Number 4 (1910) of the Carnegie Foundation for the Advancement of Teaching, New York.

Hecker, K., Read, E., Vallevand, A., et al. 2010. Assessment of first-year veterinary students' clinical skills using objective structured clinical examinations. *J Vet Med Educ*, 37, 395–402.

Hubbell, J., Savillle, W., Moore, R. 2008. Frequency of activities and procedures performed in private equine practice and proficiency expected of new veterinary school graduates. *J Am Vet Med Assoc*, 232, 42–46.

Hughes, K., Rhind, S., Mossop, L., et al. 2018. 'Care about my animal, know your stuff and take me seriously': United Kingdom and Australian clients' views on the capabilities most important in their veterinarians. *Vet Rec*, 183, 534.

Kreisler, R., Stackhouse, N., Graves, T. 2019. Arizona veterinarians' perceptions of and consensus regarding skills, knowledge and attributes of day one veterinary graduates. *J Vet Med Educ*, 47, 365–377.

Luby, C., McIntyre, K., Jelinski, M. 2013. Skills required of dairy veterinarians in Western Canada: A survey of practicing veterinarians. *Can Vet J*, 54, 267–270.

Matthew, S. M., Bok, H. G, Chaney, K. P., et al. 2020. Collaborative development of a shared framework for competency-based veterinary education. *J Vet Med Educ*, 47, 578–593.

May, S. A., Head, S. D. 2010. Assessment of technical skills: Best practices. *J Vet Med Educ*, 37, 258–265.

May, S. A. 2015. Towards a scholarship of primary health care. *Vet Rec*, 176, 677.

Michels, M., Evans, D., Blok, G. 2012. What is a clinical skill? Searching for order in chaos through a modified Delphi process. *Med Teach*, 34, e573–e581.

Miller, G. E. 1990. The assessment of clinical skills/competence/performance. *Acad Med*, 65, S63–S67.

Molgaard, L., Hodgson, J., Bok, H., et al. 2018a. *Competency-Based Veterinary Education: Part 1 - CBVE Framework*. Washington, DC: Association of American Veterinary Medical Colleges.

Molgaard, L., Hodgson, J., Bok, H., et al. 2018b. *Competency-Based Veterinary Education: Part 2 - Entrustable Professional Activities*. Washington, DC: Association of American Veterinary Medical Colleges.

Molgaard, L. K., Chaney, K. P., Bok, H. G, et al. 2019. Development of core entrustable professional activities linked to a competency-based veterinary education framework. *Med Teach*, 41, 1404–1410.

NAVMEC. 2011. *Roadmap for Veterinary Medical Education in the 21st century*. Washington, DC: North American Veterinary Medical Education Consortium.

Norcini, J., Anderson, M., Bollela, V., et al. 2018. 2018 Consensus framework for good assessment. *Med Teach*, 40, 1102–1109.

Perrin, H. C. 2019. What are employers looking for in new veterinary graduates? A content analysis of UK veterinary job advertisements. *J Vet Med Educ*, 46, 21–27.

Petersa, H., Holzhausena, Y., Boscardinb, C., et al. 2017. Twelve tips for the implementation of EPAs for assessment and entrustment decisions. *Med Teach*, 39, 802–807.

Pirkelbauer, B., Pead, M., Probyn, P., et al. 2008. LIVE: The creation of an academy for veterinary education. *J Vet Med Educ*, 35, 567–572.

Pusic, M., Boutis, K., Hatala, R., et al. 2015. Learning curves in health professions education. *Acad Med*, 90, 1034–1042.

Read, E., Hecker, K. 2013. The development and delivery of a systematic veterinary clinical skills education program at the University of Calgary. *J Veterinar Sci Technolo*, S4, 004.

Rhind, S., Baillie, S., Brown, F., et al. 2008. Assessing competence in veterinary medical education: Where's the evidence? *J Vet Med Educ*, 35, 407–411.

Rhind, S., Baillie, S., Kinnison, T., et al. 2011. The transition into veterinary practice: opinions of recent graduates and final year students. *BMC Med Educ*, 11, 64.

Royal College of Veterinary Surgeons (RCVS). 2020. Day One Competences Statement. https://www.rcvs.org.uk/document-library/day-one-competences-statement/ Accessed May 28, 2021.

Salisbury, S. K., Chaney, K. P., Ilkiw, J. E., et al. 2019. *Competency-Based Veterinary Education: Part 3 - Milestones*. Washington, DC: Association of American Veterinary Medical Colleges.

Scalese, R. J., Issenberg, S. B. 2005. Effective use of simulations for the teaching and acquisition of veterinary professional and clinical skills. *J Vet Med Educ*, 32, 461–467.

Smeak, D. 2007. Teaching surgery to the veterinary novice: the Ohio State University experience. *J Vet Med Educ*, 34, 620–627.

Smeak, D., Hill, L., Lord, L., et al. 2012. Expected frequency of use and proficiency of core surgical skills in entry-level veterinary practice: 2009 ACVS core surgical skills diplomate survey results. *Vet Surg*, 41, 853–861.

ten Cate, O. 2005. Entrustability of professional activities and competency-based training. *Med Educ*, 39, 1243–1249.

ten Cate, O., Graafmans, L., Posthumus, I., et al. 2018. The EPA-based Utrecht undergraduate clinical curriculum: Development and implementation. *Med Teach*, 40, 506–513.

ten Cate, O., Carraccio, C., Damodaran, A., et al. 2020. Entrustment decision making: Extending Miller's pyramid. *Acad Med*, online ahead of print. doi:https://doi.org/10.1097/ACM.0000000000003800.

van Melle, E., Frank, J., Holmboe, E., et al. 2019. A core components framework for evaluating implementation of competency-based medical education. *Acad Med*, 94, 1002–1009.

Welsh, P., Jones, L., May, S., et al. 2009. Approaches to defining day-one competency: a framework for learning veterinary skills. *Rev Sci Tech*, 28, 771–777.

2

Clinical Skills Curricula: How Are They Determined, Designed, and Implemented?

Jennifer Hodgson[1], Elrien Scheepers[2], and Sarah Baillie[3]

[1] *Virginia-Maryland College of Veterinary Medicine, Virginia Tech, Blacksburg, VA, USA*
[2] *Faculty of Veterinary Science, University of Pretoria, Pretoria, RSA*
[3] *Bristol Veterinary School, University of Bristol, Bristol, UK*

Box 2.1   Key Messages

- The same principles of general curricular design should be adhered to when designing or evaluating a clinical skills curriculum
- A six-step model developed by David Kern provides fundamental, yet flexible, principles of curricular design
- Student, societal, professional, and accreditation needs should be considered
- A backward design process, with initial attention to the desired outcomes, will focus curricular design
- A prioritized Day-One Competencies list and identified core Entrustable Professional Activities will further drive the design process

- Learning objectives for clinical skills must be as specific and measurable as possible
- A variety of educational methods may be used to teach clinical skills, which are not restricted to clinical skills laboratories or clinical settings
- Implementation of a clinical curriculum will depend on available resources, buy-in from stakeholders, and a properly planned management and roll-out plan
- Evaluation of the implemented clinical curriculum must be done early and repeated as needed

---

Introduction

The goal of veterinary curricula is to educate students to be optimally prepared to enter the veterinary profession with entry-level medical knowledge and appropriate mastery of an array of clinical skills (Read and Hecker, 2013; Dilly et al., 2017; Thomson et al., 2019; Duijn et al., 2020). Not only will the qualified veterinary

professional be expected to display knowledge and mastery of skills, but he or she will also have to function as part of the veterinary team, working with veterinary nursing professionals where both the veterinarian and veterinary nurse (or "vet tech") have input into patient care and treatment (Kinnison et al., 2011). Good veterinary interprofessional practice may have benefits for the practice, the individual team members, the client, and

Veterinary Clinical Skills, First Edition. Edited by Emma K. Read, Matt R. Read, and Sarah Baillie.
© 2022 John Wiley & Sons, Inc. Published 2022 by John Wiley & Sons, Inc.
Companion website: www.wiley.com/go/read/veterinary

the patient (Kinnison et al., 2014). It can, and should, be argued that this relationship between members of the professional team should be nurtured and developed from an early stage, ideally at the level of educating students. While published studies in interprofessional education interventions are sparse, it must be acknowledged that at teaching institutions where the two groups of students are educated together, opportunities for integrated curriculum design are ample and should be fostered. Even if these opportunities do not exist because of physical separation of teaching facilities, it must be kept in mind that there are many more similarities in designing clinical skills curriculum for veterinary and veterinary nursing/veterinary technology students, than there are differences. This chapter will discuss processes in the design of clinical curricula that are similar for veterinary and veterinary nursing (or veterinary technology, as called in Australia and United States) students.

The veterinary degree, perhaps more than any of the other health science degrees, poses a challenge to curricular design due to the breadth of material that must be covered, expectations of the level of competence at graduation, and the variety of career options available to veterinarians. By recognizing the close correlation between the veterinary knowledge and clinical skills also expected of newly qualified veterinary nursing professionals, it follows that near-similar challenges are posed to the design of curricula for veterinary nurses.

Despite its importance, it is easy to slip into a pattern of ad hoc curricular development with little attention to desired outcomes (Schneiderhan et al., 2018). Therefore, contemporary veterinary curricula must refocus on the fundamental knowledge, skills and behaviors required of graduates and utilize modern methods grounded in educational theory to best achieve these (Hodgson and Ilkiw, 2017).

In the broadest sense, a curriculum is defined as the totality of student experiences that occur in the educational process (Wiles, 2009), but any planned educational experience is also considered to be an example of a curriculum (Kern et al., 2016) with

this latter definition being applicable for a section of a veterinary curriculum focused on clinical skills development. Although a clinical skills curriculum would not be the totality of veterinary training, the same principles of curricular design should be adhered to when developing, or evaluating, a clinical skills curriculum for veterinarians and veterinary nurses.

There are several fundamental tenets when approaching curricular design that have been well articulated by Kern (2016): "First, educational programs have aims or goals, whether or not they are clearly articulated. Second, medical educators have a professional and ethical obligation to meet the needs of their learners, patients and society. Third, medical educators should be held accountable for the outcomes of their interventions. And fourth, a logical, systematic approach to curricular development will help achieve these ends."

To help achieve the last of these principles, Kern developed a six-step model for curricular development in medical education (Kern et al., 2016) (see Figure 2.1). This model will be used as a framework for this chapter as all the steps are equally relevant to a veterinary clinical skills curriculum, for both veterinary and veterinary nursing students, with some modifications for the different educational contexts. Further, these principles of curricular design are fundamental, yet flexible enough to yield different types of curricula in different hands, depending on the local environment and the available resources in which the clinical skills curriculum is developed.

Steps in Clinical Skills Curricular Design

Step 1: Needs Assessment and Statement

The prompts for the development or review of a clinical skills curriculum can be multifactorial including both extrinsic (e.g. accreditation) and intrinsic (e.g. student performance evaluations) factors. A needs assessment will help answer

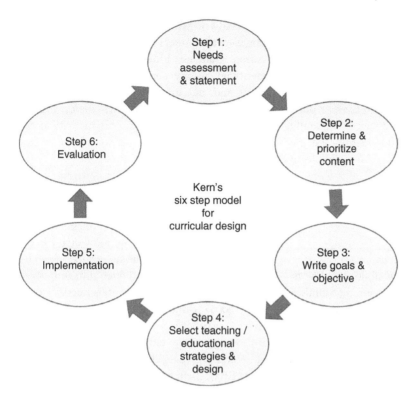

Figure 2.1 Kern's six step model for curricular design. *Source:* Based on Kern et al., 2016.

"What are you trying to achieve, why is it important, and who will benefit?" The answers to these questions should point to the distinction between the current teaching content and strategies surrounding a learning need, and what should change about it (Kern et al., 2016).

At the start, it is wise to consider whose needs are the priority. This may start with learners' needs (either skills or knowledge-based needs, readiness to learn, or time available for learning) but likely extends to the patients and communities whom the learner will be serving (Kern et al., 2016). Furthermore, when justifying changes to time or funding, an articulation of how this curriculum, or curricular change, might meet regulatory or board requirements may be useful (Schneiderhan et al., 2018). To help with this step, it may also be helpful to develop a Clinical Skills Development or Review committee, as this has been a successful strategy used by some veterinary colleges (Read and Hecker, 2013; Morin et al., 2020).

The mechanics of a needs assessment includes utilizing readily available information, as well as the collection of new information (Kern et al., 2016). The acquisition of this information can be structured (e.g. surveys), semi-structured (e.g. series of discussions with stakeholders), research/data-driven (data on learner's performance or clinical quality data) or based on regulatory requirements (Schneiderhan et al., 2018). While a needs assessment will differ between institutions, there is some information available for veterinary clinical skills that may help inform this process.

Student Needs
Feedback from faculty, staff, and veterinary and veterinary nursing students may help indicate the students' needs for clinical skills review and revision. In a recent review by Malone (2019), it was noted that while graduating students do show improvement in confidence and competence from the start of the clinical year, they

remain less than confident in many technical skills and abilities at graduation, which is echoed in other studies (Lofstedt, 2003). Similarly, only 69% of 2008 University of Queensland veterinary graduates felt satisfied with their overall skills, and only 70% felt prepared to enter practice (Schull et al., 2011). Feedback from faculty and staff may also be helpful to identify specific skills that require attention. For example, a University of Minnesota in-house survey of technicians, interns, and residents identified student challenges with animal restraint and venipuncture (Malone, 2019).

Societal and Professional Needs

The needs of clients, as well as employers, should be considered when designing a clinical skills curriculum. For example, it was shown that the majority of veterinary clients viewed technical skills (such as prioritizing patients according to illness or injury, collecting blood samples, performing a preliminary examination of an animal on admission, assisting with physical therapy techniques and making radiographs) together with emotional intelligence and professional attributes, important in the clinical practice of veterinary technology graduates with whom they interacted in the veterinary practice setting (Clarke et al., 2015). Client interviews showed that clients attached importance to graduates demonstrating professional competence, and it was therefore concluded that data such as this is useful in the design of a professional and market-driven veterinary technology curriculum (Clarke et al., 2015).

Veterinary students are licensed to practice unsupervised directly after graduation and therefore should be graduating with the knowledge and skills required to meet professional and societal demands (Greenfield et al., 2004). However, as described under student needs, many graduates do not have confidence in their own skills and abilities, which is also recognized by employers (Greenfield et al., 1997; Prescott et al., 2002; Lavictoire, 2003). In the review by Malone (2019), she described a collaboration between Banfield[*] Pet Hospitals and the University of Minnesota to identify challenges that were encountered among the 800 new small animal graduates hired each year. The survey identified surgery, dental skills, catheter placement, and venipuncture as being "critical barriers" to the success of the new graduates, leading to decreased confidence and productivity along with medical errors and increased stress to the entire team.

Lastly, Duijn et al. (2020) used entrustable professional activities (EPAs) to evaluate graduate readiness for practice. An EPA is defined as "an essential task of a discipline (profession, specialty or subspecialty) that an individual can be trusted to perform without direct supervision in a given health care context once sufficient competence has been demonstrated" (ten Cate, 2005). Duijn et al. (2020) identified five EPAs they believed were core educational objectives for veterinary curricula and surveyed new graduates regarding their readiness to perform these EPAs, including the degree of supervision they required. They found that, on average, it took graduates approximately six months until they felt ready to execute all five EPAs with distant supervision. Only after 10 months did participants feel fully competent to execute EPAs unsupervised. The authors noted that these results suggest the expectations of graduate performance may need to be nuanced but also the importance of adequate preparation of veterinarians during their education and the importance of guidance during early career to foster a successful transition from veterinary school to clinical practice. Clinical coaching of veterinary nursing students in practice is well established in certain parts of the world, but this could also be extended to veterinary nurses at the beginning of their careers to help navigating the new work environment and adapt to new situations (Kerrigan, 2018).

Accreditation Needs

There are a number of veterinary accrediting agencies worldwide, including the American Veterinary Medical Association's Council on Education (AVMA COE), the Royal College of

Veterinary Surgeons (RCVS), European Association of Establishments for Veterinary Education (EAEVE), and the Australasian Veterinary Board Council (AVBC). There is significant harmonization of accreditation standards among these organizations, with each recognizing the importance of clinical skills development within the curriculum. More specifically, Standard 9 (Curriculum) of the AVMA COE requirements states the "Curriculum must provide. . . instruction in both the theory and practice of medicine and surgery applicable to a broad range of species. The instruction must include principles and *hands-on experiences in physical and laboratory diagnostic method*s and interpretation (including diagnostic imaging, diagnostic pathology, and necropsy), disease prevention, biosecurity, therapeutic intervention (including *surgery*), and patient management and care (including *intensive care, emergency medicine* and isolation procedures) involving clinical diseases of individual animals and populations" (AVMA, 2017).

Additionally, Standard 11 (Outcomes Assessment) states "The college must have processes in place whereby students are observed and assessed formatively and summatively" on nine competencies, the majority of which include clinical skills requirements (e.g., comprehensive patient diagnosis, anesthesia, basic surgical skills, basic medicine skills, emergency and intensive care management, communication skills) (AVMA, 2017). The standard also requires colleges and schools to provide evidence of timely documentation to assure accuracy of the assessment for having attained these competencies.

Step 2: Determining and Prioritizing Content

Before a decision can be made regarding which clinical skills can, and should, be included in the curriculum, there must be a common understanding among the people involved in its implementation as to what constitutes a clinical skill in their context. For example, one study used a Delphi process and showed a marked variation between participants (British doctors involved in teaching) as to what this term meant, ranging from simple physical examination skills to include other diagnostic, communication, and practical skills (Michels et al., 2012). They concluded that acquiring clinical skills involved three components: learning how to perform certain movements (procedural knowledge), why one should do so (underlying basic and medical science knowledge or declarative knowledge), and what the findings might mean (clinical reasoning); and that these three components should be taken into account during instructional design.

Once a decision has been made as to what constitutes the range of clinical skills required for veterinary and/or veterinary nursing students to be taught in the program, the specific skills should be identified and prioritized. This may be easier said than done, as although clinical skill training is an integral part of all veterinary curricula, the specific skills that are required and how they are taught has been the subject of much debate (Malone, 2019). This is particularly the case when veterinary programs become overloaded as more and more content is added, requiring specific decisions to be made regarding the clinical skills content, as well as when and how they are taught (Malone, 2019).

Generation of a prioritized, Day-One skills list will help focus both program and student efforts on core skills, with potential additional lists that may be taught to a smaller cohort of students for colleges or schools with a tracking curriculum. These lists could be adopted from those published in the literature, and potentially modified by local practitioner input to account for regional differences (Greenfield et al., 1997). Published skills lists for veterinary students exist for general Day-One practice (Greenfield et al., 1997; Doucet and Vrins, 2009; Rush et al., 2011; Schull et al., 2011; Read and Hecker, 2013; Dilly et al., 2014; May, 2015; Kreisler et al., 2019; Malone, 2019), a variety of career paths, including those focused on small animals (Clark et al., 2002; Greenfield et al., 2004; Greenfield et al., 2005; O'Neil et al., 2014), horses

(Hubbell et al., 2008; Christensen and Danielsen, 2016), and cattle (Morin et al., 2002a; Morin et al., 2002b; Miller et al., 2004; Luby et al., 2013), as well as lists focused on specific fields such as surgery (Johnson et al., 1993; Bowlt et al., 2011; Hill et al., 2012; Smeak et al., 2012; Schnabel et al., 2013; Carroll et al., 2016; Zeugschmidt et al., 2016; Cosford et al., 2019), dentistry (Thomson et al., 2019), or theriogenology (Root Kustritz et al., 2006). Additional resources may include those skills required by accrediting agencies (e.g. the AVMA COE's 9 clinical competencies), internal surveys of faculty, and Day-One skills lists shared by other colleges (Morin et al., 2020). For veterinary nursing students, Day-One competencies lists have been published by the Royal College of Veterinary Surgeons, the Veterinary Nursing Council of Australia, and the South African Veterinary Council (RCVS 2015; VNCA 2019; SAVC 2020).

Care must be taken to prioritize these lists, as they can quickly become exhaustive, and thereby both unattainable and confusing for the student. For example, an informal survey of eight US veterinary colleges in 2009 generated a list of over 900 different, individual clinical skills, of which approximately three quarters were considered core by college faculty, but only 105 were shared by half or more of the colleges (Lizette Hardie, personal communication). Consideration, therefore, should be given to those skills considered essential for a Day-One veterinarian versus those that may be better learnt or mastered by a subset of students, or after graduation, for example in clinical practice or in continuing education programs (Malone, 2019; Duijn et al., 2020). This consideration should also take into account those skills that may be life-saving if done correctly, and those that might be life-endangering if done incorrectly (Malone, 2019). In this context, a short list of crucial skills could be valuable and could ensure we are "teaching to the common uncommonly well" (Henry J. Heinz), rather than providing exposure but not necessarily competence (Malone, 2019).

Finally, consideration should be given not only to the skills that should be included in this list, but also to the opportunities for students to master these skills. For example, the skills on a school's prioritized list of clinical skills may not be the set of skills they are exposed to in a high-level referral teaching hospital. It is essential students are given time to learn and practice these skills in the curriculum, and that this is structured to prepare them for the next stage, for example progressing from learning basic skills to more complex procedures, or in readiness for the clinical year or work placements such as extra-mural studies. Monitoring both students' confidence and competence in these skills would help ensure graduates are meeting the minimum standards expected.

Backward Curricular Design

One methodology that may help with generation of an appropriate list of core clinical skills that should be included in a curriculum is "backward design." This emerging theme in medical education has been driven by the thought that curricular design should begin at the end, rather than at the beginning (Harden, 2014). With this technique, the outcomes of the educational process are specifically determined first, then the curriculum is designed to achieve these outcomes. This is in contrast to historical approaches where the content that faculty believed should be taught was often developed at the front of the curriculum and arranged without regard for a student's ability to perform the required activities of veterinarians or veterinary nurses as a result of the teaching. A shift to competency-based education helps address this problem as this model is based on clearly defined and measurable competencies, together with student demonstration that these have been achieved. A number of competency frameworks have been developed for veterinary education, which have helped define the expected outcomes of veterinary curricula (Bok et al., 2011; Shung and Osburn, 2011; AVMA, 2017; Matthew et al., 2020; RCVS, 2020).

Entrustable Professional Activities (EPAs), Nested EPAs, and Clinical Skills

Although a focus on competencies has assisted backward curricular design, some critics of competency-based education believe that competency frameworks are too theoretical to be useful for teaching and assessment in daily clinical practice. In response to these concerns, EPAs were developed to work in tandem with competencies to produce a more "holistic" basis for curricular design (Prideaux, 2016).

An EPA is a core task which a learner can be entrusted to perform independently at a certain stage of their training when they seem ready. The EPA should be carried out within a given time frame, be observable and measurable, and allow for focused entrustment decisions (ten Cate et al. 2015), or where multiple methods exist for entrustment decisions (Duijn et al., 2019b) include the use of entrustment scales, mini-clinical evaluation exercise (mini-CEX), and direct observation of procedural skills (DOPS). In this way, EPAs operationalize observable competencies in a practical setting, because several competencies within multiple domains must be integrated simultaneously to execute the EPA (Englander et al., 2017).

Since EPAs are the routine activities that learners should be expected to perform in a clinical or workplace-based setting without direct supervision at graduation, it could be argued that these should drive curricular design for a clinical skills curriculum in the same way competencies drive curricular design and content for the entire veterinary curriculum. Recently, a number of sets of EPAs have been developed in veterinary education that focus on either core activities of graduates (Molgaard et al., 2019), those that focus on farm animals (Duijn et al., 2019a), and those that focus on surgical skills for companion animal practice (Favier et al., 2020). Additional sets of EPAs have been created for postgraduate students, such as the ones developed by Graves et al. (2020) for large animal interns.

Theoretically, an EPA can be small or simple (e.g. measuring and reporting blood pressure) or large and more complex (e.g. performing anesthesia). However, similar to the concern regarding long lists of required clinical skills, it does not make sense to develop hundreds of small EPAs resulting in long and unmanageable skills lists with no possible endpoint application. To this end, it has been suggested that smaller EPAs could be identified, which can be subsequently clustered into a large (or endpoint) EPA, where these have been called nested EPAs or sub-EPAs (ten Cate et al., 2015; Duijn et al., 2019b). In order to recognize that there are small, simple tasks or skills that need to first be mastered so that a student can be competent at the more complex EPAs, Warm et al. (2014) called these smaller units "observable practice activities" (which we call "clinical skills"), and these, in turn, can be clustered or nested into an EPA. In this way, clinical skills followed by nested EPAs can be taught and assessed in earlier years of the curriculum, allowing logical progression of skills development, as well as appropriate preparation for students to execute the larger, more complex core EPAs during their final clinical year (ten Cate, 2018). A diagrammatic representation of these relationships is outlined in Figure 2.2.

Lastly, regardless of whether competency frameworks or EPAs in tandem with competencies are used in curricular design, it is important that the required competencies (rather than individual faculty expectations) drive curricular content and the choice of logical priorities for inclusion.

Step 3: Writing Goals and Objectives

Goals are a broad overview of the content to be covered and the knowledge or skill to be obtained, while objectives are specific, measurable statements that identify the who, the what, and the when of the goal. Evidently, in a clinical skills curriculum, the focus is more on the objectives, where it is important to indicate to students the expected level of competence and how it is achieved.

As stated earlier, acquiring clinical skills includes three components: learning how to perform certain movements (procedural knowledge and abilities), why one should do these (underlying basic and clinical science knowledge), and what the findings might mean (clinical reasoning). As such, clinical skills involve more than simply performing a procedure, but clinicians

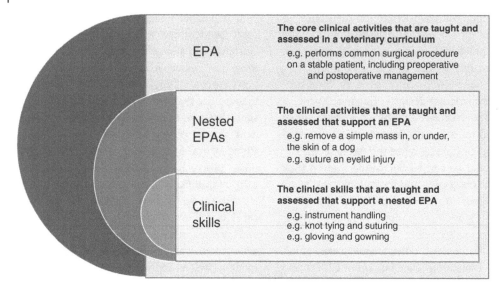

The core clinical activities that are taught and assessed in a veterinary curriculum

EPA

e.g. performs common surgical procedure on a stable patient, including preoperative and postoperative management

The clinical activities that are taught and assessed that support an EPA

Nested EPAs

e.g. remove a simple mass in, or under, the skin of a dog

e.g. suture an eyelid injury

The clinical skills that are taught and assessed that support a nested EPA

Clinical skills

e.g. instrument handling

e.g. knot tying and suturing

e.g. gloving and gowning

Figure 2.2 Relationship between EPAs, nested EPAs, and clinical skills.

are often not consciously aware of the complex interplay of different parts of a clinical skill (including knowledge and decision points) that they are practicing and accordingly do not teach all these aspects to students (see Chapter 3 for more detail) (Michels et al., 2012). When designing a clinical skills curriculum, the underpinning knowledge and the interpretation of results must be included along with the procedural knowledge and practice in the curriculum and be appropriately reflected in the learning objectives used for each component.

When writing learning objectives for clinical skills, they need to be as specific and measurable as possible and must appropriately reflect what the student "will be able to do" at the end of the learning session, with as few interpretations as possible. The verbs chosen to be used in the objective must also be relevant for each aspect of the clinical skill and reflect the learning that is hoped to be achieved. For example, if *monitoring oscillometric blood pressure in a dog* is a clinical skill that is expected of graduates, the following objectives could be appropriate, but may be located in different learning strategies (see Step 4).

At the end of the learning session, the student will be able to:

Learning objective	Skill required
Identify times when it is necessary to monitor blood pressure in a dog and the equipment needed to perform this procedure	Underpinning (declarative) knowledge
Apply a blood pressure cuff in the correct manner to the limb of a dog and read the output	Procedural skill and knowledge
Interpret the results of blood pressure readings as normal or abnormal and identify the required responses to abnormal readings	Clinical reasoning

When selecting verbs to include in learning objectives, words such as "learn," "understand," "know" or "appreciate" are vague, will be difficult to measure and should not be used (Schneiderhan et al., 2018). Additionally, verbs that imply recall of knowledge would not be appropriate for the objectives focused on procedural abilities e.g. "list," "identify," "differentiate." Better verbs for these objectives include "execute," "perform," "prepare," "calculate" etc.

Step 4: Selecting Teaching/ Educational Strategies and Design

Although we traditionally think of teaching clinical skills in a laboratory setting or in clinics, a number of different educational methods and strategies may be used to teach these skills, including lectures, laboratory classes, and flipped classroom techniques. Each of these methods has its own advantages and disadvantages in relation to teaching clinical skills. Regardless of the method selected, application of educational theory should underpin the delivery of the learning strategy. For example, teaching methods that promote active rather than passive learning should be encouraged. Active learning occurs when students engage in activities that promote analysis, reflection, and problem-solving. Further, any educational method that includes an appropriate motivational context, a high degree of student activity, interaction with peers and teachers, and a well-structured knowledge base will encourage a deep approach to learning. Conversely, any teaching method that has a heavy workload, high contact hours, excessive material, or an emphasis on coverage is likely to push students to a superficial approach to learning (Grant, 2013).

Educational Strategies
Lectures and Whole-Class Activities
Although lectures and whole-class techniques are generally less applicable for learning clinical skills, they may be an effective and efficient tool for learning if used properly. Their primary role is often information transfer, which may include the underpinning knowledge required for performing a clinical skill, understanding when a clinical skill is indicated, and how results of a procedure may be interpreted. During lectures, active learning may be encouraged with the use of classroom exercises that promote engagement, such as short quizzes using audience response systems or quick peer discussions (e.g. "Think-Pair-Share"). Alternatively, group based, clinical problem-solving activities can be planned around the whole-class activities as

described in team-based learning (Michaelsen et al., 2014). In one study, open discussion (rather than lecture) improved medical student scores on both essay and multiple choice questions regarding surgical disorders, without adding additional time (Sirikumpiboon, 2014).

Careful consideration must be given, however, when determining if a lecture regarding a clinical knowledge or skill is needed. For example, when anatomy lecture time was cut by 25% but laboratory time was spared, medical students performed similarly, despite the change in teaching hours (Petersen and Tucker, 2005).

Laboratory Classes, Including Clinical Skills Laboratories and Simulations
Laboratory classes provide necessary hands-on experiences and are essential in the development of the clinical skills required of a Day-One veterinarian or veterinary nurse. Clinical skills laboratories provide many benefits, including providing student-centered learning in a (usually) stress-free environment, supporting animal welfare, providing standardized training, and they are the ideal venues to run multi-station Objective Structured Clinical Examination (OSCE) circuits (Dilly et al., 2017). These labs provide a setting where students gain confidence and competence through deliberate and repeated practice and can receive both formative feedback and summative assessment (Morin et al., 2020). Fundamental technical skills and procedures can be taught much earlier during the curriculum than in the past, and students' technical experience at graduation will therefore not only be determined by exposure to cases encountered during final year clinical rotations, with obvious benefits on student-readiness to enter veterinary practice (Morin et al., 2020). Skills laboratories provide ample opportunities for students to learn under faculty supervision before they enter less-controlled work environments as part of their later training (Dilly et al., 2017). Furthermore, skills laboratories promote self-directed learning and peer teaching and can take advantage of new technologies and tools to enhance learning (Morin et al., 2020).

Skills laboratories are also time consuming, are often personnel-intense, and can be expensive to build and maintain, with facility development and staffing often being the largest expenses (Dilly et al., 2017). Careful consideration should be given as to how to best utilize clinical skills laboratories in order to ensure maximal efficiency of their use.

Flipped Classrooms and Additional Teaching Resources

As laboratory time is precious, it is best spent with hands-on learning. Therefore, if students can arrive ready to start practice, better utilization of the instructional team and the time available may be gained (Malone, 2019). A wide array of resources has been developed to facilitate self-directed learning, including micro-lectures that can be delivered online, learning guides, videos (including YouTube videos), audiovisual aids, and self- and peer-assessment checklists (Read and Hecker, 2013; Dilly et al., 2014; Malone, 2019; Morin et al., 2020). The information that can be included in the learning guides can comprise the name of the activity, reason the skill or procedure is important in veterinary practice, step-by-step instructions for performing the activity, descriptions of common errors, suggested resources, relevant Day-One skills, and a sample evaluation form (Morin et al., 2020). These resources are now typically combined in an online mini-course or flipped classroom for students to complete prior to the practical lab session, resulting in better preparation and use of class time (Frendo Londgren et al., 2020), and enhanced performance on OSCEs (Decloedt et al., 2020).

Videos and computer-assisted learning modules have been used successfully to teach a variety of basic, as well as advanced, clinical skills in medical education (Malone, 2019). In veterinary education, students using a self-learning computer module to learn nasogastric intubation in a horse out-performed those taught via lecture plus live demonstration as assessed through knowledge tests, time to successful intubation, and confidence levels (Abutarbush

et al., 2006). In another study, Langebaek and colleagues (Langebaek et al., 2016) evaluated which resources veterinary students used most frequently for a castration laboratory and found the students preferred videos to texts, reviewed the video repeatedly while many did not open the text documents, and recalled material from the videos better than from other sources. In a study involving veterinary nursing students, Dunne et al. (2015) found that teaching clinical skills by means of video clips and practical classes were preferred over live animal practical laboratories or demonstrations, as students felt safer with these controlled methods/environments as a first introduction to a practical procedure or clinical skill. However, in most situations the skills taught by either micro-lecture and/or video-only do not effectively substitute for time spent with hands-on training in the laboratory and are not generally sufficient as the sole method of learning clinical skills (Malone, 2019).

Curricular Design

In addition to the methods used to teach in a clinical skills curriculum, consideration should also be given to how these are placed in the overall curriculum. For example, are clinical skills best taught in stand-alone courses, or should they be integrated in other courses within the curriculum? Furthermore, should skills be taught in a stepwise manner or in an intensive training block?

Stand-Alone Courses or Integrated into Existing Courses

Clinical skills may be taught as stand-alone courses or their instruction may be integrated into existing ones, and there is no evidence to suggest that one design is better than the other. Regardless of the type of course in which they are taught, it is important to map where, and potentially how, these skills are taught, as well as when and how they are assessed. Furthermore, there should be a logical sequence to skill development that aligns with building toward the final level of clinical competence that has been determined as being core for a curriculum.

An additional advantage to curricular mapping is that it allows identification of material that is included, as well as any uncoordinated or unplanned repetition. Mapping may also identify skills that may be redundant, irrelevant, or unsuitable for a Day-One veterinarian or veterinary nurse.

Spiral (Distributed) versus Block (Intensive) Training
Most skills programs describe a spiral curriculum, where skills are taught in a stepwise building fashion and become more complex at each iteration, providing reinforcement and integration (Harden, 1999; Malone, 2019). For example, early laboratories may concentrate on basic animal handling skills to ensure students can safely work with the range of species they are likely to encounter later in their training and in the eventual workplace. For clinical skills, initially individual items such as surgical scrubbing and gloving are the focus, while over time these skills are added together to develop procedural competence. In this way, patient preparation, surgeon and assistant scrubbing and gloving, and patient draping can be combined to simulate the initial steps of surgery (Malone, 2019). Furthermore, this progression may include advancing from the use of low-fidelity models to the use of high-fidelity models to the use of live animals (Read and Hecker, 2013; Carroll et al., 2016).

Spiral training usually takes place over an extended time frame (e.g. months to years) and is an iterative process, with practice of the basic procedures often preceding addition of new procedures. Taught this way, multicomponent skills can be broken into parts and practiced either sequentially or in random order (Malone, 2019), and this is the most common method currently employed in veterinary education (Read and Hecker, 2013; Carroll et al., 2016).

An alternate model is to teach all the skills required for a procedure in an intensive block of time, as has been described in medical education (Gershuni et al., 2013). This method is often used in postgraduate professional development training due to its time efficiency (Malone, 2019). In one study in medical education, a distributed training program for suturing skills was compared to intensive block training where the distributed program included more practice opportunities and resulted in better skills retention (Gershuni et al., 2013).

Step 5: Implementation

The implementation phase can be divided into several different steps, starting with the identification of resources. Resources fall into four basic categories that include personnel, time, facilities, and funding (Kern et al., 2016). Utilizing existing resources (faculty and staff already employed, educational materials already developed, time already put aside in a curriculum, rooms already dedicated to teaching) can lower costs and increase likelihood of success (Schneiderhan et al., 2018).

Resources
Personnel
Personnel involved in teaching or supporting a clinical skills laboratory may include teaching faculty (including residents, interns, graduate students, and adjunct faculty), staff (including licensed veterinary nurses, technical and administrative support), and information technologists (if needed for computerized modules). The number of people in each of these categories is highly variable between institutions depending on the teaching load and the availability of facilities and equipment. However, it is now common practice to have a supervisor and/or director of the facility, which may be full- or part-time faculty appointment, as well as a manager, which is frequently a full- or part-time staff appointment (Morin et al., 2020). Staffing needs may be inconsistent depending on the timing of the laboratory sessions, the number of students being taught, and the proximity to assessments. Therefore, it may be preferable to have multiple part-time personnel and fewer full-time personnel.

Sufficient staffing by competent, approachable teachers coupled with readily accessible resources for self-directed learning are critical to the success of a clinical skills laboratory (Dilly et al., 2017).

Veterinarians who have been in primary care practice and experienced veterinary technicians can be good instructors for Day-One skills (Morin et al. 2020), while peer- or near-peer teaching has also been used to help staff their clinical skills laboratories (Baillie et al., 2009; Read and Hecker, 2013; Bates et al., 2016; Carroll et al., 2016; ten Cate et al., 2018).

Time

Time is often one of the most precious resources and includes the time required for the students, as well as the time of the teachers, including faculty and staff (Schneiderhan et al., 2018). The amount of time reported for teaching clinical skills in veterinary curricula is highly variable. For example, at the University of Minnesota, laboratory training (including nonclinical skills training) comprises 13–15% of the curriculum depending on the student's track (Malone, 2019). Others report having had to cut core laboratory hours and replace these with optional sessions (Carroll et al., 2016). In contrast, another program reported reducing didactic content in years 1 and 2 by 25%, which enabled them to add clinical practical courses focused on fundamental clinical skills (Morin et al., 2020). Similarly, the University of Calgary, with a very strong emphasis on clinical skills training, reports 20% of the curriculum devoted to skills training (Read and Hecker, 2013). Regardless of the time allocated in a program to teach these skills, it is often necessary to have creative and efficient training of clinically appropriate knowledge and skills given the constraints on available time in the curriculum (Thomson et al., 2019).

An additional consideration when allocating time for a clinical skills curriculum is how students should progress. Most professional programs move students through training programs as cohorts in a time-based manner. However, students enter a professional curriculum with vastly different backgrounds, experiences, innate abilities, and interests. Conversely, students may leave a program with a different set of skills depending on their rate of learning and their area of interest (e.g. track). Does it make sense to assume students should progress at the same speed and need the same learning opportunities, particularly with the high cost of laboratory teaching (Malone, 2019)?

The corollary to this concept is a curriculum that focuses on competency (i.e. time independent), which is one of the fundamental tenets of competency-based medical curricula (ten Cate et al., 2018). However, given the current administrative restrictions for veterinary programs, this could be difficult to achieve for individual students. A possible alternative would be to offer those students demonstrating proficiency in a given core set of skills opportunities to learn additional, more advanced skills and for these to be acknowledged through a portfolio or "badging" system and which could be used to enhance employability. This approach could be utilized in earlier years of the curriculum, as well as during the clinical years.

Facilities

Facilities are the spaces such as classrooms or clinic sites where the learning will take place (Schneiderhan et al., 2018). Laboratory spaces that are dedicated to teaching clinical skills are becoming increasingly common in veterinary education (Read and Hecker, 2013; Dilly et al., 2014; Dilly et al., 2017). These facilities allow students to practice a range of professional and technical skills in a safe and nonconfrontational environment, before performing them in "real-world" settings such as a veterinary teaching hospital. Furthermore, many models and simulations are now available to assist the learning in this environment and are discussed at length in other chapters in this book. Other venues where clinical skills may be taught include university farms, teaching hospitals, external affiliated practices, and a wide range of agricultural and veterinary premises during extramural studies.

Funding

Funding for a clinical skills curriculum should include all the direct financial costs and faculty compensation, as well as any other hidden costs (Schneiderhan et al., 2018). Annual budgets for clinical skills training are highly variable among veterinary programs but can run into the hundreds of thousands of dollars if all costs are included. In determining an appropriate budget for a clinical skills curriculum, careful consideration should be given not only to the costs for development of the curriculum but also the ongoing costs of personnel and equipment for teaching activities, as well as assessments to ensure its sustainability.

Buy-in

The next step in implementation is obtaining support internally from stakeholders to the curriculum, and at times externally when funding or support for other resources is needed (Schneiderhan et al., 2018). Stakeholders are those most directly impacted by implementation of a clinical skills curriculum and may include students, the faculty who are responsible for the teaching, as well as administrative personnel (e.g. Dean of the College). Having their support and enthusiasm is crucial to the success of any curriculum.

External support may become necessary when resources beyond what is available to the program or school are needed, either financially or in terms of facilities, and has been described in a number of veterinary programs (Morin et al., 2020).

Management Plan and Roll Out

The final phases in this step are the design of a management plan and roll out. The management plan should detail the actual step-by-step process of how the curriculum will be delivered and include the who, what, where, and how for each component or teaching strategy, as well as anticipating where any barriers might arise during the roll out of the curriculum (Schneiderhan et al., 2018). Some of these barriers may be anticipated in advance, along with a plan to mitigate them.

The last step in implementation is the actual roll out. Before this occurs, it may be helpful to initially pilot sections of the clinical skills curriculum to enthusiastic stakeholders, both to gain more support and to identify and rectify any barriers to implementation so that the odds of success are increased (Schneiderhan et al., 2018). This pilot can be followed by a phasing-in, where new portions are added until the full curriculum is ultimately implemented.

Step 6: Evaluation

The final step in the curricular design process is evaluation. This is a process of determining the merit, value, or worth of a program that has been implemented (Kern et al., 2016). Although evaluation is often considered to be the final phase of curriculum development, it should span the entire process and is often cyclical and iterative. Furthermore, evaluation of a curriculum should be conducted early on, or at key points, in order to inform changes and identify opportunities for improvement. Alternatively, evaluations can be made after full implementation to determine whether a curriculum was successful, and for whom, in order to report back to stakeholders (Schneiderhan et al., 2018).

The major steps of a curricular evaluation involve five components, which will be discussed briefly below.

1: Develop a clear plan to use evaluation results
Although it may seem counterintuitive, the first step of an evaluation is to consider who will use the evaluation results and how they will be used. An evaluation that is never used will not be worth the effort (Schneiderhan et al., 2018). A utilization plan should include a dissemination plan (e.g. written reports, presentations, discussion sessions) and the specific audience for each. In addition, the utilization plan should detail what types of actions may be anticipated based on the results; for example, could the report lead to changing, ending, or expanding the clinical skills program?

2: Determine how to measure objectives
The next step is to determine how to measure the outcomes of the learning objectives for the curricular initiatives and whether these were met by the students. This step mostly incorporates

assessment and includes consideration of the different assessment strategies that are most appropriate to assess student learning of clinical skills, as well as the timing of these assessments, whether they will be repeated, and what ultimately demonstrates proficiency for more complex clinical activities that incorporate multiple competencies and skills.

3 & 4: Collect and analyze data

Data collection might involve tests, interviews with students or instructors, performance assessments, or other methods (Schneiderhan et al., 2018). Analyzing pre-post differences can be particularly helpful in assessing whether learning has been enhanced (or otherwise) due to curricular changes.

5: Use evaluation results by applying lessons learnt

The final step is to use the evaluation results and apply lessons learnt to the curriculum (Kern et al., 2016). Guided by the utilization plan, this step consists of disseminating information to relevant stakeholders and making use of the results to improve learning outcomes or the learning experience. This evaluation process should also be iterative as educators apply lessons learnt and then subsequently evaluate and implement further improvements to the curriculum.

Conclusions

The education of veterinary and veterinary nursing students so they are optimally prepared to enter the veterinary profession with entry-level veterinary knowledge and appropriate mastery of many clinical skills can be achieved by starting with the precise design of both theoretical and clinical skills curricula. In essence, the end result should be an integrated curriculum. This becomes more obvious if it is considered that the same principles of theoretical curriculum design are also applied to the design of a clinical skills curriculum.

By conducting a needs analysis and statement, identifying and prioritizing content, and formulating a clinical skills program in a backward design process, a curriculum that will educate students in aspects of applied knowledge, clinical skills, and clinical reasoning can be produced. A clinical skills curriculum can be successfully implemented depending on resources. It is vital that the newly implemented curriculum is assessed and subsequently improved. If the steps and processes described in this chapter are followed, the clinical curriculum design process will be focused and simplified, with a resultant well-prepared qualified veterinarian and veterinary nurse.

References

Abutarbush, S. M., Naylor, J. M., Gale Parchoma, G., et al. 2006. Evaluation of traditional instruction versus a self-learning computer module in teaching veterinary students how to pass a nasogastric tube in the horse. *J Vet Med Educ*, 33, 447–454.

American Veterinary Medical Association. 2017. Council on Education Accreditation Policies and Procedures: Requirments [Internet]. 2017 Sept, 2017 [cited 2020 Jan 2] Accessed January 2, 2020.

Baillie, S., Shore, H., Gill, D., et al. 2009. Introducing peer-assisted learning into a veterinary curriculum: A trial with a simulator. *J Vet Med Educ*, 36, 174–179.

Bates, L. S. W., Warman, S., Pither, Z., et al. 2016. Development and evaluation of vetPAL, a student-led, peer-assisted learning program. *J Vet Med Educ*, 43, 382–389.

Bok, H. G. J., Jaarsma D. A. D. C., Teunissen, P. W., et al. 2011. Development and validation of a competency framework for veterinarians. *J Vet Med Educ*, 38, 262–269.

Bowlt, K. L., Murray, J. K., Herbert, G. L., et al. 2011. Evaluation of the expectations, learning and competencies of surgical skills by undergraduate veterinary students performing canine ovariohysterectomies. *J Sm Anim Pract*, 52, 587–594.

Carroll, H.S., Lucia, T. A., Farnsworth, C. H., et al. 2016. Development of an optional clinical skills laboratory for surgical skills training of veterinary students. *J Am Vet Med Assoc*, 248, 624–628.

Christensen, B. W., Danielsen, J. A. 2016. Utility of an equine skills course: A pilot study. *J Vet Med Educ*, 43, 406–419.

Clark, W. T., Kane, L., Arnold, P. K., et al. 2002. Clinical skills and knowledge used by veterinary graduates during their first year in small animal practice. *Aust Vet J*, 80, 37–40.

Clarke, P. M., Al-Alawneh, L., Pitt, R. E., et al. 2015. Client perspectives on desirable attributes and skills of veterinary technologists in Australia: Considerations for curriculum design. *J Vet Med Educ*, 24, 217–231.

Cosford, K., Hoessler, C., Shmon, C. 2019. Evaluation of a first-year veterinary surgical skills laboratory: A retrospective review. *J Vet Med Educ*, 46, 423–428.

Decloedt, A., Franco, D., Martlé, V., et al. 2020. Development of surgical competence in veterinary students Using a flipped classroom approach. *J Vet Med Educ* (adv. online). https://doi.org/10.3138/jvme.2019-0060.

Dilly, M., Tipold, A., Schaper, E., et al. 2014. Setting up a veterinary medicine skills lab in Germany. *GMS Zeitschrift fur Medizinishe Ausbildung*, 31, Doc20.

Dilly, M., Read, E. K., Baillie, S. 2017. A survey of established veterinary clinical skills laboratories from Europe and North America; present practices and recent developments. *J Vet Med Educ*, 44, 580–590.

Doucet, M. Y., Vrins, A. 2009. The importance of knowledge, skills, and attitude attributes for veterinarians in clinical and non-clinical fields of practice: a survey of licensed veterinarians in Quebec, Canada. *J Vet Med Educ*, 36, 331–342.

Duijn, C. C., ten Cate, O., Kremer, W. D. J., et al. 2019a. The development of entrustable professional activities for competency-based veterinary education in farm animal health. *J Vet Med Educ*, 46, 218–224.

Duijn, C. C., van Dijk, E. J., Mandoki, M., et al. 2019b. Assessment tools for feedback and entrustment decisions in the clinical workplace: A systematic review. *J Vet Med Educ*, 46, 340–352.

Duijn, C. C., Bok, H., ten Cate, O., et al. 2020. Qualified but not yet fully competent: Perceptions of recent veterinary graduates on their day-one skills. *Vet Rec*, 186, 216.

Dunne, K., Brereton, B., Bree, R., et al. 2015. Integrating customised video clips into the veterinary nursing curriculum to enhance practical competency training and the development of student confidence. *AISHE-J*, 7, 2581.

Englander, R., Frank, J. R., Carraccio, C., et al. 2017. Toward a shared language for competency-based education. *Med Teach*, 39, 582–587.

Favier, R. P., Godijn, M., Bok, H. G. J. 2020. Identifying entrustable professional activities for surgical skills training in companion animal health. *Vet Rec*, 186, 122.

Frendo Londgren, M., Baillie, S., Roberts, J. N., et al. 2020. A survey to establish the extent of flipped classroom use prior to clinical skills laboratory teaching and determine potential benefits, challenges, and possibilities. *J Vet Med Educ*, e20190137. doi: https://doi.org/10.3138/jvme-2019-0137. Online ahead of print.

Gershuni, V., Woodhouse, J., Brunt, M. L. 2013. Retention of suturing and knot-tying skills in senior medical students after proficiency-based training; results of a prospective, randomized trial. *Surgery*, 154, 823–830.

Grant, J. 2013. Principles of curriculum design. In: *Understanding Medical Education; Evidence, Theory and Practice*. Swanwick, T. (ed.). London, UK: Wiley-Blackwell. pp. 31–46.

Graves, M. T., Castro, J. R., Anderson, D. E. 2020. Veterinary intern program for entrustable professional activities skills, a.k.a. intern boot camp. *J Vet Med Educ*, 47, 321–326.

Greenfield, C. L., Johnson, A. L., Klippert, L., et al. 1997. Employer-based outcomes assessment of recent graduates and comparison with performance during veterinary school. *J Am Vet Med Assoc*, 211, 842–849.

Greenfield, C. L., Johnson, A. L., Schaeffer, D. J. 2004. Frequency of use of various procedures, skills, and areas of knowledge among veterinarians in private small animal exclusive or predominant practice and proficiency expected of new veterinary school graduates. *J Am Vet Med Assoc*, 224, 1780–1787.

Greenfield, C. L., Johnson, A. L., Schaeffer, D. J. 2005. Influence of demographic variables on the frequency of use of various procedures, skills, and areas of knowledge among veterinarians in private small animal exclusive or predominant practice and proficiency expected of new veterinary school graduates. *J Am Vet Med Assoc*, 226, 38–48.

Harden, R. M. 1999. What is a spiral curriculum? *Med Teach*, 21, 141–143.

Harden, R. M. 2014. Progression in competency-based education. *Med Educ*, 48, 838.

Hill, L. N., Smeak, D. D., Lord, L. K. 2012. Frequency of use and proficiency in performance of surgical skills expected of entry-level veterinarians by general practitioners. *J Am Vet Med Assoc*, 240, 1345–1354.

Hodgson, J. L., Ilkiw, J. 2017. Curricular design, review, and reform. In: *Veterinary Medical Education: A Practical Guide*. Hodgson, J. L., Pelzer, J. M. (eds.) Hoboken, NJ: Wiley-Blackwell. pp. 3–23.

Hubbell, J. A. E., Saville, W. J. A., Moore, R. M. 2008. Frequency of activities and procedures performed in private equine practice and proficiency expected of new veterinary school graduates. *J Am Vet Med Assoc*, 232, 42–46.

Johnson, A. L., Greenfield, C. L., Klippert, L., et al. 1993. Frequency of procedure and proficiency expected of new veterinary school graduates with regard to small animal surgical procedures in private practice. *J Am Vet Med Assoc*, 202, 1068–1071.

Kern, D. E., Thomas, P. A., Hughes, M. T. 2016. *Curriculum Development for Medical Education: A Six-Step Approach*. Baltimore: Hopkins University Press.

Kerrigan, L. 2018. Coaching and mentoring: Beyond the role of the clinical coach in veterinary practice. *Vet Nurse*, 9, 70–74.

Kinnison, T., Lumbis, R., Orpet, H., et al. 2011. Piloting interprofessional education interventions with veterinary and veterinary nursing students. *J Vet Med Educ*, 38, 311–318.

Kinnison, T., May, S. A., Guile, D. 2014. Inter-professional practice: From veterinarian to the veterinary team. *J Vet Med Educ*, 41, 172–178.

Kreisler, R., Stackhouse, N., Graves, T. 2019. Arizona veterinarians' perceptions of and consensus regarding skills, knowledge, and attributes of day one veterinary graduates. *J Vet Med Educ*, 47, 365–377.

Langebæk, R., Nielsen, S. S., Koch, B. C., et al. 2016. Student preparation and the power of visual input in veterinary surgical education: An empirical study. *J Vet Med Educ*, 43, 214–221.

Lavictoire, S. 2003. Education, licensing, ad the expanding scope of veterinary practice members express their views. *Can Vet J*, 44, 282–284.

Lofstedt, J. 2003. Confidence and competence of recent veterinary graduates--is there a problem? *Can Vet J*, 44, 359–360.

Luby, C., McIntyre, K., Jelinski, M. 2013. Skills required of dairy veterinarians in Western Canada: A survey of practicing veterinarians. *Can Vet J*, 254, 267–270.

Malone, E. 2019. Evidence-based clinical skills teaching and learning: What do we really know? *J Vet Med Educ*, 46, 379–398.

Matthew, S. M., Bok, H. G. J., Chaney, K. P., et al. 2020. Collaborative development of a shared framework for competency-based veterinary education. *J Vet Med Educ*, 47, 578–593.

May, S. A. 2015. Towards a scholarship of primary health care. *Vet Rec*, 176, 677–682.

Michaelsen, L. K., Davidson, N., Major, C. 2014. Team based learning practices and principles in comparison with cooperative learning and problem based learning. *J Excell Coll Teach*, 25, 3–15.

Michels, M., Evans, D., Blok, G. 2012. What is a clinical skill? Searching for order in chaos through a modified Delphi process. *Med Teach*, 34, e573–e581.

Miller, R. B., Hardin, L. E., Cowart, R. P, et al. 2004. Practitioner-defined competencies required of new veterinary graduates in food animal practice. *J Vet Med Educ*, 31, 347–365.

Molgaard, L. K., Chaney, K. P., Bok, H. G. J., et al. 2019. Development of core entrustable professional activities linked to a competency-based veterinary education framework. *Med Teach*, 41, 1404–1410.

Morin, D. E., Constable, P. D., Troutt, H. F., et al. 2002a. Surgery, anesthesia, and restraint skills expected of entry-level veterinarians in bovine practice. *J Am Vet Med Assoc*, 221, 969–974.

Morin, D. E., Constable, P. D., Troutt, H. F., et al. 2002b. Individual animal medicine and animal production skills expected of entry-level veterinarians in bovine practice. *J Am Vet Med Assoc*, 221, 959–968.

Morin, D. E., Arnold, C. J., Hale-Mitchell, L. K., et al. 2020. Development and evolution of the clinical skills learning center as an integral component of the Illinois veterinary professional curriculum. *J Vet Med Educ*, 47, 307–320.

O'Neil, D. G., Church, D. B., McGreevy, P. D., et al. 2014. Prevalence of disorders recorded in dogs attending primary-care veterinary practices in England. *PLoS One*, 9, e90501.

Petersen, C. A., Tucker, R. P. 2005. Undergraduate course work in anatomy as a predictor of performance: comparison between students taking a medical gross anatomy course of average length and a course shortened by curriculum reform. *Clin Anat*, 18, 540–547.

Prescott, J., Hagele, W. C., Leung, D., et al. 2002. CVMA task force on "education, licensing, and the expanding scope of veterinary practice". *Can Vet J*, 43, 845–854.

Prideaux, D. 2016. The emperor's new wardrobe: The whole and the sum of the parts in curriculum design. *Med Educ*, 50, 3–23.

RCVS. 2020. Day One Competences. https://www.rcvs.org.uk/document-library/day-one-competences Accessed May 28, 2021.

Read, E. K., Hecker, K. G. 2013. The development and delivery of a systematic veterinary clinical skills education program at the University of Calgary. *J Veterinar Sci Technolo*, 4, S4, 004.

Root Kustritz, M. V., Chenoweth, P.J., Tibary, A. 2006. Efficacy of training in theriogenology as determined by a survey of veterinarians. *J Am Vet Med Assoc*, 229, 514–521.

Royal College of Veterinary Surgeons. 2015. Day-One Competences for Veterinary Nurses. https://www.rcvs.org.uk/document-library/day-one-competences-for-veterinary-nurses/ Accessed May 28, 2021.

Rush, B. R., Biller, D. S., Davis, E. G., et al. 2011. Web-based documentation of clinical skills to assess the competency of veterinary students. *J Vet Med Educ*, 38, 242–250.

Schnabel, L. V., Maza, P. S., Williams, K. M., et al. 2013. Use of a formal assessment instrument for evaluation of veterinary student surgical skills. *Vet Surg*, 42, 488–496.

Schneiderhan, J., Guetterman, T. C., Dobson, M.L. 2018. Curriculum development: A how to primer. *Fam Med Community Health*, 7, e000046.

Schull, D. N., Morton, J. M., Coleman, G. T., et al. 2011. Veterinary students' perceptions of their day-one abilities before and after final-year clinical practice-based training. *J Vet Med Educ*, 38, 251–261.

Shung, G., Osburn, B. I. 2011. The North American Veterinary Medical Education Consortium (NAVMEC) looks to veterinary education for the future. Roadmap for veterinary medical education in the 21st century: responsive, collaborative, flexible. *J Vet Med Educ*, 38, 320–327.

Sirikumpiboon, S. 2014. Comparison of didactic lectures and open-group discussions in surgical teaching. *J Med Assoc Thai*, 97, S140–144.

Smeak, D. D., Hill, L. N., Lord, L. K., et al. 2012. Expected frequency of use and proficiency of core surgical skills in entry-level veterinary practice: 2009 ACVS core surgical skills diplomate survey results. *Vet Surg*, 41, 853–861.

South African Veterinary Council. 2020. Vet Nurses SAVC Day 1 Skills. https://www.savc.org.za/pdf_docs/2020_H_VET_NURSES_SAVC_Day_1_Skills_v3_FINAL.pdf Accessed May 28, 2021.

ten Cate, O. 2005. Entrustability of professional activities and competency-based training. *Med Educ*, 39, 1176–1177.

ten Cate, O., Chen, H. C., Hoff, R. G., et al. 2015. Curriculum development for the workplace using entrustable professional activities (EPAs): AMEE guide no. 99. *Med Teach*, 37, 983–1002.

ten Cate, O. 2018. A primer on entrustable professional activities. *Korean J Med Educ*, 30, 1–10.

ten Cate, O., Gruppen, L. D., Kogan, J. R., et al. 2018. Time-variable training in medicine: Theoretical considerations. *Acad Med*, 93, S6–S11.

Thomson, A., Young, K. M., Lygo-Baker, S., et al. 2019. Evaluation of perceived technical skills development by students during instruction in dental extractions in different laboratory settings - a pilot study. *J Vet Med Educ*, 46, 399–407.

Veterinary Nursing Council of Australia, VNCA. 2019 Day-One Competency Standards. https:// www.vnca.asn.au/vnca-day-one-competency-standards/ Accessed May 28, 2021.

Warm, E. J., Mathis, B. R., Held, J. D., et al. 2014. Entrustment and mapping of observable practice activities for resident assessment. *J Gen Intern Med*, 29, 1177–1182.

Wiles, J. 2009. *Leading Curriculum Development*. Thousand Oaks, CA: Corwin Press, p. 175.

Zeugschmidt, E., Farnsworth, C. H., Carroll, H. S., et al. 2016. Effects of an optional clinical skills laboratory on surgical performance of third-year veterinary students. *J Am Vet Med Assoc*, 248, 630–635.

3

How Are Clinical Skills Taught?

Sarah Baillie[1], Matt R. Read[2], and Emma K. Read[3]

[1] *Bristol Veterinary School, University of Bristol, Bristol, UK*
[2] *MedVet, Worthington, OH, USA*
[3] *College of Veterinary Medicine, The Ohio State University, Columbus, OH, USA*

Box 3.1   Key Messages

- Carefully plan and structure a clinical skills class to ensure the learning objectives are achieved

- Teaching in the clinical workplace can be challenging. Apply sound educational techniques to enhance learning opportunities

- Adopt and use evidence-based methods for teaching clinical skills (e.g. George and Doto's 5-steps)

- Use questioning and feedback for successful clinical skills teaching that will promote learning

- Experts are not always the best teachers because they practice in a highly automated manner. Utilize cognitive task analysis (or at least be aware of what it informs us about experts) to help identify the details that students need to know and to create better learning guides (e.g. do not only include step-by-step actions, but include relevant procedural knowledge and decision points as well)

- Students benefit from separation of knowledge input and hands-on skills practice or demonstration to avoid cognitive overload. Avoid giving verbal feedback while the student is performing a skill. Instead, ask them to focus on what you are saying first, then allow them to practice again

---

Introduction

There have been many advances in clinical skills teaching in veterinary medicine in recent years, aided by the introduction of clinical skills laboratories (Dilly et al., 2017), a more structured approach within the curriculum (Read and Hecker, 2013) and more widespread adoption of associated faculty development programs (Warman et al., 2015).

The traditional approach to learning that many veterinarians will have experienced as students themselves followed Halstead's apprenticeship model for training surgeons (Halsted, 1904). This involves the trainee observing an expert performing an operation or procedure ("see one"), performing the same procedure under supervision ("do one"), and eventually being the person instructing another trainee ("teach one").

Veterinary Clinical Skills, First Edition. Edited by Emma K. Read, Matt R. Read, and Sarah Baillie.
© 2022 John Wiley & Sons, Inc. Published 2022 by John Wiley & Sons, Inc.
Companion website: www.wiley.com/go/read/veterinary

This teaching model has been used for many years, but the modern clinical workplace presents a number of challenges for both teachers and learners that make it difficult to adhere to this formula. These include time pressures, increasing cohort size, the impact of specialization (i.e. case suitability), and finding opportunities to learn (Scalese and Issenberg, 2005; Smeak, 2007; Luhoway et al., 2019). Since there are many changes and challenges, it is timely to reflect upon our approaches to teaching clinical skills to ensure students are taught in ways that effectively and efficiently equip them with the skills they will require.

Clinical skills are taught throughout the veterinary curriculum, and approaches typically include a combination of animal handling sessions on farms, at stables, etc., and hands-on classes in a clinical skills laboratory. These experiences are designed to prepare students for learning during subsequent workplace-based experiences such as in a teaching hospital or other type of clinical setting. Individual component skills are taught first (e.g. knot tying and suturing), equipping the learner with the "building blocks" that will enable them to later perform procedures that comprise multiple skills together (e.g. performing a surgical operation on a cadaver or operating on a live patient).

The following sections describe techniques for teaching clinical skills, including preparing for and structuring a session and adopting established teaching and learning methods. Although many of the examples are used in the context of teaching in a clinical skills laboratory, they may be equally relevant and applied to workplace-based settings. Particular challenges related to teaching in a busy clinic and the differences between the teacher (the expert) and the student (a novice) will also be discussed.

Techniques for Teaching Clinical Skills

Preparation for Teaching

> By failing to prepare, you are preparing to fail.
>
> *Benjamin Franklin.*

Preparation before any teaching event is key to the delivery of a successful learning activity. In certain clinical settings, teaching will make use of clinical cases that are encountered as part of daily practice and is therefore somewhat opportunistic. However, when running scheduled practical classes in a clinical skills laboratory, there is a series of preparatory steps that should be undertaken prior to the session (Dent and Hesketh, 2004). Start by taking time to become familiar with the students' existing knowledge and their stage in the curriculum, including reviewing related teaching (e.g. lectures and previous practicals) and any material students will be able to access as part of their preparation (e.g. flipped classroom videos, instruction booklets, quizzes) (Frendo Londgren et al., 2020). The learning outcomes for the session need to be appropriate for the stage of the curriculum in order to build on prior learning and prepare students for the next stage. The number of skills and length of the session also need careful consideration. In an individual session, "less is more" and emerging evidence suggests that shorter, more frequent sessions may be beneficial to learning (Malone, 2019). Attention also needs to be given to how the class will be run, including the layout of the room, what equipment and supplies will be needed, what technology will be needed, how subgroups of students will be managed (e.g. appropriate size of groups for the activity), and the anticipated duration of individual activities (a visible clock or audible timer can be helpful for ensuring all outcomes are achieved within the allotted time).

Use of a template for planning the learning activity can be useful (see Figure 3.1) and should include all of the details for the class preparation and teaching delivery. Following the learning activity, notes can be made about how closely the experience matched the plan and what changes will need to be made before delivering the same lesson in the future (e.g. a week, a month, or a year later). In this way, use of templates can be very helpful for both experienced teachers, as well as those who are new to teaching a particular lesson. Using standardized

Practical plan template (example)

Practical class details

Name of class:	*Basic surgical skills*	Duration:	*2 hours*
Instructors (n):	2	Names	...... , ...
Student year:	Vet 2	Group size:	18

Stations (*list stations if multiple skills/stations being taught at same time*)
- Station 1: Suturing Skills (using silicon pad)
- Station 2: Suturing Skills (using tea-towel)
- Etc.

Room layout (*example*)

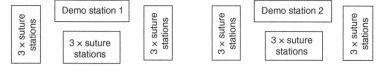

Learning objectives
- Place a simple interrupted suture
- Place a cruciate suture
- Place continuous suture pattern
- Remove sutures

Introduction (*by the practical class lead*)

Welcome the students to the practical class, introduce the teaching team, explain aims (learning objectives) and provide other information e.g. describe any biosecurity and/or health & safety consideration, explain groupings and timings, divide students into groups, etc.

Teaching details (*information for each station/skill/instructor*)

Text description providing detailed instructions that demonstrator follows: Demonstrate how to perform [skill]; describe steps, common mistakes...

Equipment list (for each station)

Item	No. required	Present ✔
Silicon suture pad	9	
Tea towel suture model	9	
Suture material [detail: type, size]	2 reels nylon, 3-0	
Instrument A	18	
Etc.		

Timings (*if rotating round different stations include a timetable*)

Station	1st 60 minutes	2nd 60 minutes	*Add column/s and*
1	Group A	Group B	*row/s if there are*
2	Group B	Group A	*more groups*

Notes:

Figure 3.1 A template for practical class preparation, set up, and delivery.

templates also encourages a more consistent approach to teaching for practical classes throughout the curriculum, making it easier for students to prepare for learning sessions and set their expectations appropriately.

Structuring the Session and Learning Outcomes

As with other types of teaching activity, clinical skills sessions should follow a predefined structure. It can be tempting to simply "jump-in" and start teaching, but adopting and adhering to a defined structure ensures that the objectives will be clear to the learners and helps the teacher design and deliver a successful session. For example:

1) Start the session by setting the scene. Consider using a "bridge" or "hook" to engage the students with the topic and set the stage in terms of why the skills that will be learned that day are important and relevant. This may include discussing a case that was recently seen in the teaching hospital or referring to a previous lab session where related skills were first presented. The introduction may also involve some sort of formal or informal assessment ("pretest") to gauge the students' level of preparation prior to the session in order to learn where the cohort is starting in terms of knowledge and ability.

2) Explain the objectives or learning outcomes for the session. The best objectives are SMART (Specific, Measurable, Attainable, Relevant, Time-oriented). Make the objectives "learner-focused" and outline what skills will be taught using "action words"/ verbs. Consider following the template of "By the end of this session, you will be able to. . .." Write the objectives in terms of *WHO, does WHAT, under WHAT conditions.*

3) Teach the skill(s). The session should be designed to encourage participatory learning with all students being engaged in each of the learning objectives.

4) At the end of the session, perform a formal or informal assessment ("posttest") to see how much the students learned and whether or not they have achieved the objectives as outcomes (i.e. can they perform the skills at the expected level?).

5) Summarize the session and let the students know what they can expect to learn next time and what they can do to prepare. Wrap up the session on time.

When setting relevant learning objectives in different contexts, it is useful to consider Bloom's taxonomy (1956) and the three "learning domains" – cognitive, affective, and psychomotor. The *cognitive* domain has been described as training the doctor (or veterinarian) as a scientist and scholar and is probably the most familiar domain (Tomorrow's Doctors, 2009). In this case, learning objective verbs are chosen to align with the six different levels that progress from basic recall to higher order problem-solving and clinical reasoning skills (e.g. from low to high – "list, explain, demonstrate, compare, evaluate, develop"). The *affective* (or behavioral) domain trains the doctor or veterinarian as a professional and relates to their ability to receive, respond, value, and organize. Learning objective verbs for this domain might include "listen, notice, express, choose and consider". The *psychomotor* domain trains the doctor or veterinarian as a clinician. This domain relates specifically to hands-on or "doing" (i.e. clinical skills), so verbs for this domain might include "observe, identify, locate, practice, prepare, design, produce, and perform".

Considering any one of the domains in isolation is an oversimplification as all three are used when learning clinical skills, especially in a workplace setting or clinical situation. However, when teaching in a clinical skills laboratory, the psychomotor domain is arguably the most relevant, and learning objectives are typically written using context-specific "doing" verbs (e.g. *apply* a headcollar; *catch* and *turn* (restrain) a sheep; *place* a simple interrupted suture pattern; *perform* a complete physical examination, *find* and correctly *identify* the bovine uterus). Often, there needs be an associated adjective or adverb in order to make the objective more specific and, potentially, more measurable and time-oriented (e.g. tie a *square* knot *securely*). The number of learning objectives needs to be achievable in the session (i.e. how many skills can realistically be taught and learned in the allotted time?) and should be set at an appropriate level for the stage in the curriculum.

Adopting an Established Teaching Method

There are several established techniques that may be used to optimize the teaching of clinical skills. These include a four-step approach (Walker and Peyton, 1998 – described further in Chapter 8) and George and Doto's (2001) five-step method that is explained in detail below (Table 3.1).

George and Doto's Five-Step Method for Teaching Clinical Skills

Step 1: Conceptualization. Initially, the instructor needs to explain the relevance of the skill in a clinical context and the importance of learning to perform the skill correctly. When teaching basic surgical skills such as suturing, students will usually already be aware of the relevance of the skill to clinical work, though not necessarily. More importantly,

students may not be familiar with the criteria that define success or the consequences of poor technique, so these must be explicitly stated. For surgical skills, these include and relate to:

- maintaining sterility throughout the procedure, how and when common mistakes are made, recognizing hazards (developing situational awareness);
- benefits of handling instruments correctly;
- knot tying and the importance for effective hemostasis;
- appropriate placement of the suture in relation to the wound edges;
- correct suture tension (neither too tight or too loose) and the consequences for wound healing.

It is important to always include the conceptualization step. Don't just rush in and start demonstrating the skill or students will learn it out of context.

Step 2: Visualization. The next step involves a silent demonstration of the skill so that the learner can observe every step of the skill or procedure once through, from start to finish. This allows the learner to focus on developing a mental image of the entire skill (which will serve as a reference both during their own learning and when they reflect on their own performance), and gives them a sense of how

Table 3.1 The five-step method for teaching clinical skills.

Step	Action by instructor and/or learner
1. Conceptualization	Instructor explains why the skill is important to ensure that learner understands (i.e. it is clear).
2. Visualization	Instructor demonstrates performance of the skill silently while learner observes
3. Verbalization	Instructor repeats their demonstration of the skill while explaining each step (verbalizing as well as demonstrating). Learner watches and listens and may ask questions for clarification.
4. Verbalization	Learner repeats back (describes) the steps to instructor. Instructor provides feedback/corrections.
5. Performance	Learner practices skill. Instructor provides feedback.

Source: Based on George and Doto, 2001.

long it should take to successfully perform the skill once mastery is obtained. Additionally, this step allows the learner to only use one of their five senses (or "channels" – in this case, *visual*), rather than trying to concurrently process extra information through an additional channel (e.g. *auditory*), whereby they would have to integrate a visual image with a verbal description at the same time.

Setting expectations is also important. Inform the learner that Step 2 involves the instructor first demonstrating the procedure silently (and explain why. . .), otherwise it may feel like a strange way for them to be taught.

Step 3: Verbalization (by the instructor). The instructor then repeats their demonstration of the skill, while this time also slowly and deliberately verbalizing each step of the skill or procedure for the learner (see discussion of CTA-based instruction below). Verbalization helps to ensure that the learner is aware of all the steps, allowing them to arrange the steps in the correct sequence and to develop a narrative. It also allows the learner to process the information using more than one channel at a time, when they are more likely to benefit from it. At the end of Step 3, the instructor should pause and ask if the learner has questions, requires any clarification, or would like any part of the demonstration or explanation repeated.

Step 4: Verbalization (by the learner). The learner then describes the steps of the skill or procedure back to the instructor, thereby demonstrating their knowledge (recall) of the skill, as well as the organization or sequencing of the steps. The instructor provides clarification and feedback, and the learner may repeat the description (or parts of it) if required. Step 4 provides an opportunity for informal assessment of the cognitive levels of Miller's pyramid of clinical competence (i.e. "Knows" and "Knows how") (Miller, 1990).

Step 5: Performance. Lastly, the learner performs the skill by themselves while being observed by the instructor who provides feedback and additional guidance as required. The "performance" step will need to be repeated by the learner, as mastery depends on repetitive and deliberate practice (Ericsson, 2004). Repetition may occur during the initial learning session (as the student is learning the skill for the first time), either supervised or self-directed at a later date (in order to consolidate the skill or prepare for an assessment such as an OSCE) or strategically to reinforce the skill (e.g. prior to a workplace-based experience or clinical rotation).

Practical Considerations

Adhering to the five-step method may sometimes seem difficult, especially in a large practical class or when teaching in a busy workplace setting. However, being familiar with George and Doto's method (or an equivalent technique, e.g. Walker and Peyton, 1998, see Chapter 8) and applying it wherever possible is strongly recommended. In situations where a student is struggling to learn and perform a skill, explicitly following these steps is more likely to result in a better outcome for the learner.

The importance of including the *conceptualization* stage cannot be overstated. For example, bandaging may seem like it would be an easy skill to learn, or students may consider it to be irrelevant to their career if they have never observed a veterinarian performing the skill. For this reason, including a demonstration that emphasizes the importance of good technique and the consequences of poor technique will enhance "conceptualization" and improve learner focus during the class.

There are also opportunities to delegate some of the five steps to the learner or a peer. Part or all of Steps 1–3 may be incorporated into flipped classroom materials, so more time can be used for hands-on practice and provision of instructor feedback during the in-person teaching session (Frendo Londgren et al., 2020). The flipped classroom approach is gaining more widespread adoption in veterinary education (Matthew et al., 2019), partly because the associated technology has become easier for teachers to use to create online material. In the flipped component, students undertake self-directed learning in preparation for the face-to-face class (e.g. watch videos of skills or procedures, view short voiceover presentations, and self-assess using quizzes). Another option, particularly when working with large groups, is to use a peer-to-peer approach at Step 4, with one student recalling (verbalizing) the steps to another student who uses an instruction booklet to check accuracy and sequence, referring to the instructor for clarification if required.

Using Questions to Enhance Learning

Using questions appropriately can enhance the teaching session and improve learning (Edmunds and Brown, 2010). Questions can be used at the start of a practical class or clinical case to gather information that enables the teacher to pitch a session at the right level (e.g. serving as an informal "pretest" to establish what the students already know, their prior experience and skill level, specific concerns, and areas to focus on). As described in the Calgary-Cambridge model, effective communication with patients or clients involves using a combination of open-ended and closed-ended questions, and a similar approach should be used between teacher and learner when considering a clinical skill (Kurtz et al., 1998). There is often a tendency for instructors to use closed-ended questions, especially when they are busy (e.g. Have you auscultated the heart before? Have you found the uterus?), whereas use of open-ended questions will elicit more useful information (e.g. Can you tell me what you are finding difficult? Can you show me. . .?). Open-ended questions are typically perceived as being less judgmental and help to establish a more constructive environment for learning.

Effective use of questions can help to engage students more actively in their own learning. Sometimes, having a predetermined set of questions that may be applicable to all students is useful, especially since the same "pain points" often recur in every session with more than one student. Being prepared with well thought-out questions can lead to more effective teacher–student

interactions and more efficient use of time. Additionally, consideration should be given to how to respond to incorrect answers using a constructive approach. Finally, it is important to give the student time to think and answer the question. Counting to five silently to oneself can be helpful to avoid the temptation to simply jump-in with the correct answer or to reframe the question or ask a different question too quickly.

Providing Useful Feedback

Feedback is integral to the learning process and is an important consideration when teaching clinical skills in practical classes and in a clinical setting (Issenberg et al., 2005; McGaghie et al., 2010). The provision of *specific, owned, accurate, timely,* and *constructive* feedback by the teacher enables the student to learn from, and during, an activity (Molloy and Boud, 2013). The feedback that is received is crucial in informing the student's preparation for the next activity (e.g. another attempt at performing the same skill), progressing to the next level, or planning for the next case. Without feedback, the student may not know what was done well, they may not be aware of errors in performance, and they may not be able to accurately focus on areas for future improvement. Therefore, in addition to confirming what has been done correctly, the teacher should identify where the learner's performance has not yet achieved the desired objectives, describe the differences between observed and desired performance, determine possible reasons for the differences, and then work with the learner to formulate a plan on how to improve.

Building feedback into all teaching activities is crucial for learning, but finding the time and opportunity is sometimes difficult (e.g. in a large group setting or when dealing with the many demands of a busy clinical workplace). Practicing providing feedback, setting aside dedicated time (especially in a workplace setting), and normalizing the process will help to embed good practice. In a clinical skills laboratory, there may be opportunities to build in peer-to-peer feedback, with the feedback provider using pre-prepared materials such as a skills instruction booklet as a guide. Feedback is discussed in more detail in Chapter 5.

Understanding Learning Preferences of Students

Each individual tends to use slightly different approaches to learning and will have preferences for one or a subset of styles. In the context of teaching and learning clinical skills, the visual-auditory-reading-kinesthetic (VARK) model can be quite useful to help frame learner preference (Barbe and Milone, 1981; Fleming, 1995; Ramani and Leinster, 2008). In VARK, visual learning (V) involves *seeing* (e.g. observing a procedure or watching a video), auditory learning (A) involves *hearing* (e.g. listening to a history being taken or a description of how to perform a skill by a teacher or over a podcast), reading/writing learning (R) involves *text* (e.g. reviewing the content of an instruction booklet or lab manual prior to a Clinical Skills lab), and kinesthetic learning (K) involves hands-on *doing* (e.g. performing a physical examination, tying a knot). In any group of learners, there will be different preferences represented, which may or may not align with that of the teacher or the modality most easily used for a particular setting. Usually, most adult learners are able to adapt their preferred learning preference to a given situation and use a variety of approaches, depending on the circumstances. However, for example, if a student who is having difficulty in a clinical skills lab prefers to read about the skill and process that information first, simply repeating a visual demonstration of the skill over and over may not help that particular learner in that moment. In such a situation, pausing to ask about a student's particular learning preference and then giving the student time to process the same information using their preferred format may lead to a better learning outcome.

Using Educational Theories
Cognitive Load Theory

Cognitive load theory was first described in 1988 and focuses on three different memory systems used by learners: *sensory*, *working*, and *long-term* memory (Young et al., 2014). Based on this theory, large volumes of information enter a student's mind via the "sensory memory" system where it is retained for a very short period of time (i.e. milliseconds) before some of the information is raised to the level of "working memory." Working memory can only process up to seven elements of information at one time and, as such, may become a bottleneck when the brain is busy processing certain items into "long-term memory." Long-term memory is essentially limitless, however, the information must be "chunked" into pieces and "tagged" so that it is easier to retrieve later.

Cognitive load theory suggests that students have separate channels for perceiving and processing *auditory*, *visual*, and *tactile* information and that large volumes of such information are received via the sensory memory with most of what is perceived not being raised to the level of conscious awareness. During learning, the student has to filter out "irrelevant" stimuli while screening in "relevant" information, which means that working memory has a profound impact on the rate of actual learning (Young et al., 2014). As the learner progresses through the various stages of learning (i.e. from novice to expert – see Table 3.2), they tend to be better able to cope with an increasing amount of information at any one time and their ability to multitask improves. According to cognitive load theory, the purpose of instruction is to help organize and store increasing amounts of complex knowledge into the long-term memory (Kalyuga and Sweller, 2018).

Dual Process Theory

Dual process theory is often discussed alongside cognitive load theory and explains how information is processed and how patterns are recognized (see Figure 3.2). Dual process theory states that novice learners are not able to adequately recognize patterns and draw conclusions from them, therefore they rely primarily on "Type 2 thinking" which is slow, analytical, and highly reliable (Kahneman, 2011). Therefore, novice

Table 3.2 Characteristics of novice to expert.

Stage of learning	Characteristics
Novice	Task needs to be deconstructed into context-free steps that are presented with a single method. Components of skills must be taught and practiced slowly and individually. Teaching needs to be provided in a distraction-free environment.
Advanced beginner	Teacher can add in situational components, where the student is given examples of the context that the skill is used in and how it can be modified accordingly. Slight variations in skill techniques may be introduced.
Competence	Student values reward when task is done well and specific feedback to help get them "back on track" when they are struggling. Learner commits to "learning better" and reflects on their progress (holistic thinking). Student demonstrates capability and can blend skills together.
Proficient	Student acts more independently. Student thinks intuitively rather than analytically, and quickly knows what is necessary to achieve learning goals. There is emphasis on the small details to show greater efficiency in performance. Able to perform with other distractions occurring in the environment.
Expert	Student has knowledge and gains experience to apply that knowledge. Exhibits automated decision-making and intuitively knows what needs to be done to correct their performance so results are almost always flawless. Practices deliberately to improve performance.

Source: Based on Dreyfus, 2004.

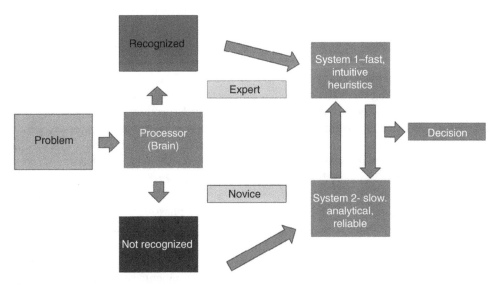

Figure 3.2 Dual process theory.

learners need to be deliberate in their learning and are unable to handle multiple cognitive channel inputs at one time. They often desire "one right answer" and want details to be explained to them in simple, black-and-white terms. Alternatively, experts predominantly rely on pattern recognition and form correct solutions most of the time. Unlike novices, experts are able to perform tasks automatically with very little mental effort and use Type 1 thinking, which is intuitive, fast, and relies on heuristics ("short cuts") (Kahneman, 2011). In addition, Type 1 and Type 2 systems not only operate parallel to each other, but they also toggle back and forth between each other (Young et al., 2014).

It is important to remember that novices are not only learning new skills, they are also learning to coordinate between the two different types of processing information. As such, teaching delivery requires adaptation depending on how advanced the students are and what learning characteristics they are displaying. How much toggling between Type 1 and Type 2 thinking actually occurs often depends on the experience of the individual and their amount of accumulated expertise. Experts seemingly know when to slow down and pay attention to the little details to solve complex problems and can determine individual solutions to situations that do not follow the normal pattern (Moulton et al., 2010; Kahneman, 2011). Learner progression allows for greater reliance on intuitive thinking and less need for slower contemplation because the learner has memories of that motor skill already stored.

Dual process theory helps explain why the most successful and widely used teaching models for clinical skills are those that support "limited input to novice students" via "one channel at a time," affording them the opportunity to deliberately mentally process what they are being exposed to in "measured doses" (George and Doto, 2001).

Novice students and clinicians who experience increasing cognitive load too early in the learning process find this interferes with their ability to perform hands-on skills (e.g. novice surgeons in the operating room listening to music have reported that their technical performance suffers compared to peers in a more distraction-free space) (El Boghdady and Ewalds-Kvist, 2020). In most training environments, there is an almost continual flow of information from the more experienced clinician to the novice trainee, and this can be challenging for the student's learning, acting as both a blessing and a curse (Young et al., 2014). Verbal feedback is useful for improving performance, but too much feedback while a novice learner is

actively trying to work can lead to cognitive overload and result in more errors. Suspending performance of a technical skill while receiving verbal information such as feedback can result in the novice being better able to later recall the information that was provided to them and improves their ability to assimilate that information with the technical skill that was being practiced (Young et al., 2014). In summary, novices work hard to learn, and the more we can optimally focus their learning during practice sessions, the more quickly they will progress.

Encouraging Deliberate Practice

The mastery of any skill requires practice, whatever the context. Just as a professional athlete will repeatedly practice the most important aspects of their sport or a musician will puts in many hours of rehearsal prior to a performance, students who are learning clinical skills should be no different (Kneebone, 2009). Teachers are responsible for ensuring that their students are aware of the need for repeated practice and of the resulting benefits for consolidating learning, addressing areas of weakness (identified through feedback), and maintaining their skills. However, not all time spent practicing is equal. Practice should be *deliberate*, *purposeful*, and *focused*, which requires both opportunity and time (Ericsson, 2004; McGaghie et al., 2011). Initially, encouraging deliberate practice is more important than emphasizing speed (Norman et al., 2018). "Get good first, get fast later" is a phrase sometimes used in surgical training to emphasize this point.

Practice also depends on motivation, which may be based on the student's desire to become a proficient clinician (i.e. "intrinsic motivation"), an imminent assessment such as an OSCE (i.e. "extrinsic motivation"), or a combination of both. A clinical skills laboratory provides an ideal environment for students to practice and may be enhanced by an open-door policy and/or scheduled revision sessions (Dilly et al., 2017; Morin et al., 2020). When students practice, guidance on their performance of the skill should be available from an instructor or by referring to a video or instruction booklet. In the workplace, clinical teachers have an important role in identifying the opportunities for practice and encouraging students to engage in these learning activities (Ramani and Leinster, 2008). Students also need to appreciate the importance of seeking expert feedback to avoid incorrect technique continuing unchecked. This enables the learner to reflect on their ability and develop a plan for further practice and improvement.

Making the Most of a Clinical Setting

The techniques described in the previous sections are applicable to both practical classes in a clinical skills laboratory and in a clinical setting. Compared to the controlled and somewhat artificial setting of a teaching laboratory, the clinical workplace is truly authentic. As such, it provides numerous and diverse opportunities for students to learn new skills and practice existing ones and typically involves integration of clinical skills (technical/procedural) with communication and clinical reasoning. However, the clinical workplace also poses challenges to both the teacher and the learner (Irby and Bowen, 2004; Ramani and Leinster, 2008). Clinicians need to juggle the roles of both care provider and teacher, often while under time and financial pressures. In addition, the environment is not always suitable for teaching, learning, or giving feedback (e.g. when a client is present). Consideration needs to be given to case suitability, welfare of the patient, and the needs of other members of the team. Not surprisingly, students may be anxious about entering the workplace and their associated emotions, and stress may not be conducive to learning (Langenbæk et al., 2012).

The challenges of teaching in the modern clinical workplace have driven some of the recent changes in veterinary curricula. For example, clinical skills training has become embedded earlier and more comprehensively in the curriculum in attempt to improve student preparation for work placements and clinical rotations (Read and Hecker, 2013; Morin et al., 2020). There are specific tips and approaches to assist those teaching alongside their clinical work (Ramani and Leinster, 2008). The way learners perceive the clinical teacher is an important factor in their success. In addition to being clinically competent, positive characteristics include enthusiasm for teaching, being organized and clear, targeting teaching to the learner's needs, and creating an environment conducive to learning by empowering learners, developing rapport, being approachable, and modeling self-evaluation and reflective practice (Irby and Papadakis, 2001; Ramani and Leinster, 2008). Effective clinical teachers prioritize teaching whenever possible, identify and optimize learning opportunities for their students, act as role models, and habituate teaching within their daily practice (Smith and Kohlwes, 2011).

Clinicians can use similar techniques to classroom-based teachers, including preparation and planning, setting expectations, explaining learning objectives, using appropriate questions, providing feedback, and encouraging self-directed learning and practice (Irby and Bowen, 2004). Specific strategies have been described for use in the clinical setting and becoming familiar with such approaches can be helpful when juggling the demands of the workplace (Irby and Bowen, 2004; Ramani and Leinster, 2008; Vanka and Hovaguimian, 2019). One example of a strategy that can be used by an instructor on the clinic floor is the "One-minute preceptor," which aims to enable clinicians to capitalize on teaching opportunities while acknowledging the short time available (Neher et al., 1992). There are five steps or "microskills" that make up this teaching strategy (see Box 3.2).

Overall, there will always be a balance between clinical commitments and finding time and suitable opportunities to teach. An educator's enthusiasm and passion for teaching as well as their efficiency and efficacy in promoting learning can be optimized through having an awareness of different teaching techniques and strategies, understanding the relevant parts of the curriculum (e.g. the learners' level of skill and experience), engaging in

Box 3.2 The 5-Step "One-Minute Preceptor."	
1) Getting a commitment	Learner is encouraged to engage from the start (e.g. to suggest a diagnosis or to perform a procedure), rather than the clinician providing the answer or performing the skill
2) Probing for supporting evidence	Learner is asked to describe their reasoning (e.g. justify the diagnosis or treatment plan). Sometimes called a "think-aloud" technique. Clinician provides feedback
3) Teach a general principle	Clinician identifies the most relevant aspects of the current case for the leaner and generalizes to other similar situations
4) Reinforce what was done well	Clinician provides feedback on the positives ("Part 1" – what went well), ensuring that the feedback is specific and informs the way the learner should prepare their plan for the next case/encounter/activity
5) Give guidance about errors and omissions	Clinician provides feedback on the negatives ("Part 2" – opportunities for growth). This should be phrased constructively and the teacher should encourage the learners to self-assess and engage in reflection

Source: Based on Neher et al., 1992.

ongoing faculty development, and modeling the qualities of being a reflective practitioner.

Using a Flipped Classroom

It is increasingly common for students to complete an online module as a "flipped classroom" prior to a clinical skills session. An example of this could be providing high-quality supporting learning resources (e.g. instruction booklets and video demonstrations) prior to a clinical skills lab, enabling students to make the most of their supervised hands-on practical time. To this end, there are numerous open-access resources such as clinical skills videos (Müller et al., 2019) and booklets (Bristol Veterinary School, 2017). To be used effectively, flipped classroom resources should focus on teaching core knowledge (e.g. identifying instruments) and/or the steps of a skill (e.g. placing a simple interrupted suture). They should be short and include materials that reflect different learning styles (e.g. videos, images, short voiceover presentations, quizzes) (Frendo Londgren et al., 2020). There are several benefits to using this approach, including the fact that students will come to the lab better prepared, students will be more engaged in the lesson, students will use class time more effectively, and instructors can focus on teaching the skills and providing feedback rather than starting at the beginning with all of their learners (Decloedt et al., 2020; Frendo Londgren et al., 2020). However, teachers should not underestimate the time required to design a flipped classroom (Moffett, 2015). Adopting a standard template (a "storyboard") can be helpful and the associated technologies are becoming easier to use. The practical class lead should ensure all instructors are familiar with the resources, as well as emphasize the importance of doing the preparation to students.

Peer Observation of Teaching

Another way that instructors can enhance their clinical skills teaching is to engage in "peer observation of teaching," a valuable and constructive process where teachers seek feedback from peers, which subsequently helps them reflect upon and improve their teaching skills (Siddiqui et al., 2007). Peer observation may be part of the institution's educational quality assurance or may be initiated by an individual who is interested in receiving objective and non-judgmental feedback on their teaching. The relationship may continue if both parties are willing to revisit the process again in the future.

The peer-observation process typically involves three stages: (i) a *pre-observation* meeting between the observee and the observer to discuss the aims of the observation, the context of the lesson, and any specific areas that the observee is interested in receiving focused feedback on; (ii) the *observation* itself, where the observee delivers their lesson and the observer watches and makes notes of what they see; and (iii) a *post-observation* debrief (usually not immediately following the lesson) where the observer provides their feedback and the observee shares their own reflections and thoughts. During the debrief meeting, plans to refine the lesson and/or goal setting for the observee's future teaching may also be made.

There are a number of benefits to peer observation, including providing an opportunity to share ideas about best practice, to discuss and solve dilemmas with a colleague, and to encourage engagement in reflective practice (Newman et al., 2019). In the context of clinical skills teaching, the observer could be asked, for example, to provide specific feedback on the teacher's overall management of the lesson (e.g. Were all students able to keep up and achieve the stated learning outcomes? How was the timing of the session? Were other instructional team members used effectively? Was the room layout conducive to learning?).

Cognitive Task Analysis Techniques to Inform Skills Teaching

By now, it should be obvious that teaching technical skills is challenging for both teachers and learners. To achieve optimal effectiveness, skills should be taught in a detailed, step-by-step, standardized, analytical fashion that allows in-depth comprehension of the essential elements of the technique by a student (Velmahos et al., 2004). However, merely describing *what* to do assumes that the learner has the background knowledge and skill to know *how* to do it (Sullivan et al., 2008). This is not always the case, and most learners are often reluctant to ask for further instruction or clarification in order to not appear unprepared or unintelligent.

The term "task analysis" refers to the process of determining the individual steps that comprise a given task and how these steps are structured and relate to one another (Johnson et al., 2006). This type of evaluation has been used in a variety of industries and may be performed for a variety of reasons, including use as an educational resource or to identify potential safety issues. Basic (e.g. behavioral) task analysis focuses on documenting the obvious, observable movements and actions that someone makes in order to achieve a goal or complete a task, and has been commonly used when teaching and assessing students. However, when a procedure is complex or requires decisions to be made along the way (i.e. many of the clinical skills taught and learned in veterinary medicine), a more detailed mapping of the operator's thought process is required to fully understand and describe how they successfully complete the task (Johnson et al., 2006).

"Cognitive task analysis" (CTA) is an extension of traditional task analysis and is particularly valuable when expert knowledge and decision-making contribute to the successful completion of a task. In addition to documenting the observable steps that are performed sequentially to complete the task (e.g. those that simple task analysis might identify), CTA uses in-depth interviews and discussions with experts to identify the cognitive skills or mental demands that are needed to solve difficult problems and perform complex procedures (Campbell et al., 2011). As such, CTA is a unique educational method that can be used to deconstruct the automated skills of experts and accelerate the learning curve of novices when it comes time to learn such complex cognitive skills for themselves (Sullivan et al., 2007). For these reasons, CTA is ideal for informing and enhancing the teaching and learning of clinical skills.

CTA is especially useful for documenting sophisticated performance expertise in situations where complex *overt* (i.e. observable) actions are linked with many *covert* (i.e. non-observable) decisions that support them. This is especially relevant to procedures that have "unsighted" components (e.g. rectal palpation), where it is not necessarily possible for a teacher to demonstrate their physical movements to a student or provide a student with accurate feedback on their own performance (Low-Beer et al., 2011). In these situations, CTA can be very useful for identifying and describing an expert's knowledge, including the unconscious automated components, by deconstructing the task into its constituent steps and considerations. More than simply documenting *what* you can see someone doing, CTA allows you to understand *how* they do it and *why* they do what they do.

Across various studies, instruction that involves CTA-based teaching materials have been shown to enhance learning when compared to traditional teaching methods. Because CTA is based on several experts' opinions and experiences, students have access to (and can benefit from) a wider, more objective breadth of knowledge than they would if they learned solely under one supervisor (Luker et al., 2008). For example, medical students that were taught how to perform central venous catheterization using CTA-derived instruction were more likely to perform the procedural steps correctly, required less attempts and less direction when performing the skill and had fewer complications (Velmahos et al., 2004). In other studies, learners in the CTA-groups had better technical competence one- and six months following their instruction, performed better during "think out loud" assessments, outperformed control group students on procedural knowledge, and reported significantly higher self-efficacy scores (Sullivan et al., 2007; Campbell et al., 2011).

Although there are dozens of different ways to conduct CTA, typically the process is achieved by having a small number of experts formally complete a task or procedure silently while being video-recorded. Then, the same experts repeat the task for a second time (while again being recorded) with instructions to verbally articulate all of the knowledge that they require, to explain the steps that they perform, and to describe the decisions that they make. A transcript is made of the recordings and the actions that the experts described are compared with the actions that were observed in both of the videos (Read and Baillie, 2013). Following this, a semi-structured interview with each expert is conducted in order to clarify what steps are needed and what thinking was taking place during the activity. Multiple experts can be compared with one another and consensus sought across a number of individuals. A "gold standard" document is then produced and can be provided to learners as a learning tool to help them formally recognize and learn all of the important aspects of the skill, including the decision-making points that are frequently left out of the initial demonstration (Read and Baillie, 2013). The learning tool can also be used to help formulate a checklist for assessment (e.g. an OSCE) (Read et al., 2016).

At its simplest, CTA may involve interviewing at least two experts, whereby a focused and detailed description of each technical step is generated by one expert and then is validated by a second expert (Velmahos et al., 2004). Others report that three or four experts are needed for CTA to develop the "gold standard," balancing the capture of critical information with the amount of time and effort that is required in order to obtain it (Yates et al., 2012). CTA can be time consuming, and this has been noted as a detractor in applying this technique to everyday teaching and learning. It has been reported to take up to 30–40 hours to completely document one hour of expertise (Sullivan et al., 2007; Sullivan et al., 2008). Regardless of whether or not a complete CTA is undertaken to help develop learning tools for a procedure, several key take-home messages from the literature are relevant to both teachers and students.

Advice for Teachers

"Declarative knowledge" refers to *what* someone knows about facts, events, and objects and is found in our conscious working memory. "Procedural knowledge" refers to knowing *how* to perform a task and includes both motor and cognitive skills (Sullivan et al., 2008). As teachers, we need to be able to pass on both types on knowledge to our students, and this can be harder than it looks. Procedural knowledge tends to be automated and operates outside of conscious awareness (Sullivan et al., 2008). Once a skill is automated, it can be fine-tuned, so the operator can run on autopilot and execute the skill faster than conscious processes. This means that the expert omits steps and decision points while they are teaching the procedure because they have literally lost access to behaviors and cognitive decisions that are being made during execution of the skill.

In many fields, structured checklists are used to help teach and create standardized curricula for their students (Sullivan et al., 2008; Campbell et al., 2011). Typically, these checklists focus on the simple step-by-step performance of a skill, with little to no consideration of the underlying decisions that need to be made along the way. As explained above, failure to include all the cognitive steps is often the result of the people who develop the checklists being experts themselves, whereby "automated knowledge" is achieved after years and years of practice and experience, and the basic elements of a task are no longer performed with any level of conscious awareness (see Figure 3.3). In other words, although experts are reasonably good at accurately describing what it is they can already be observed doing by someone else (i.e. step-by-step performance of a skill), they have great difficulty articulating the decisions they make while performing the procedure because their procedural knowledge has largely become automated (Yates et al., 2012). The information that would

make this obvious is no longer accessible to conscious processes, so content experts – the very people who are often the ones developing the teaching materials and doing the teaching – will inadvertently omit many steps when trying to describe how to perform a procedure, leaving their students without all of the critical information they need to know about a task (Sullivan et al., 2008; Campbell et al., 2011; Read and Baillie, 2013). Studies have shown that when experts are asked to recall or teach a complex procedure or task that they perform routinely, they unintentionally omit 50–70% of the information that someone would need to learn in order to perform the task successfully (Sullivan et al., 2008; Smink et al., 2012; Yates et al., 2012).

By either using CTA itself to develop teaching materials, or simply being aware of what CTA explains about experts as teachers, an instructor will be in a much better place when it comes to assisting students.

A teacher will never be able to teach everything they need to teach about a subject matter in the time available with students in class. More importantly, they will likely be unable to articulate over half of what a student needs to learn and will likely teach different students different things depending on what they may ask or what the instructor thinks to correct while observing them perform the skill.

CTA can be used to develop and enhance teaching materials so that students can more effectively prepare prior to attending their clinical skills lab (i.e. flipped classroom-style) and allows for delivery of a more consistent approach to student learning overall. Students will be able to obtain the relevant basic technical knowledge ahead of time and also learn the standardized method that they will subsequently use to perform the procedure in person. As described above, to effectively reach the widest audience possible for this style of instructional delivery, the teacher should ideally develop several types of learning tools that present the same information to students with different learning styles (e.g. written manuals, short videos, podcasts). No matter what type of tool is developed, the information presented must be standardized. This allows trainees to learn the basic principles and techniques of the procedure, as well as the essential decision points ahead of time, so they can focus on learning the nuances of the technique during the face-to-face learning session, rather than the instructor needing to start from the beginning. Students in the teaching lab can therefore spend their time honing their knowledge and skills, allowing them to use their time with the expert more efficiently (Luker et al., 2008; Sullivan et al., 2008).

When putting together lessons, instructors should focus not only on the declarative ("what") knowledge that can be tested by use of traditional methods such as MCQs, true or false questions, OSCE stations, etc., but they should also focus on the procedural knowledge used when performing the skill ("how," "why"). In order to speed up the learning curve, students need to be provided with as much of what an experienced instructor has learned over years of practice as possible. Why risk patient injury and force students to make the same mistakes over and over similar to when their instructor was developing expertise? Why not avoid those mistakes to begin with?

To help students, an instructor needs to be deliberate. First, they should watch and record a colleague performing the same procedure they will be teaching. Next, they should review it with them in order to ask them why they completed the individual steps in the way they did. Ask about the visual and tactile cues used to make decisions, anticipating the sort of things that might go wrong, and the mistakes they have seen novices make. It can also be useful to have someone watch and record the instructor doing the procedure as well and to debrief with them too. Bottom line, an expert needs to step away from being an automated expert and free themselves up to think about why they do things the way they do, and what information they use to make decisions. Any instructor going through this process will undoubtedly enhance their teaching materials and become more aware of areas to focus their students' attention on.

CTA-based curricula can also be used for development of assessment methodology for skills certification (e.g. OSCEs) and to validate simulator models that are developed. For example, if a model cannot be used to learn the majority of the critical steps in a procedure (not just the step-by-step observable ones, but also the ones that require a decision to be made), it is probably not a very good model and likely only teaches part of the skill. Even worse, it may impart bad habits that will be hard to break later.

Advice for Students

Students should take advantage of what has been learned about the use of CTA and not only focus on the "*whats*" of a clinical skill, but on the "*hows*" and the "*whys*" as well. If, after reviewing the teaching materials that have been prepared, the student feels as though they are only being taught the basic observable steps that are used to perform a procedure, they should feel comfortable asking their teachers why the steps are performed in that order, why the teacher does things the way they do, what would happen if a particular step was performed differently or out of order, etc. Students should not be shy about asking for more information. In most cases, the instructor probably has a very good reason for doing something the way they do and trying to teach it that way, but at this point in their career the task has likely become automated and they may have not even thought about it in terms of remembering to tell their students why.

This is especially important when it comes to making decisions and teaching someone else how to make them. Most instructors do a reasonable job teaching the basic step-by-step performance of a procedure since it is easy for a student to watch them do it and then try to repeat it for themselves (e.g. the first few steps in George and Doto's approach to teaching clinical skills, discussed above). Where many teachers really fail is linking the skill to the declarative knowledge that students already have (e.g. making the skill relevant in terms of background information) and articulating the

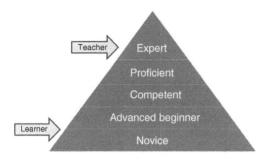

Figure 3.3 The challenge of the teacher (expert) and the learner (typically novice or advanced beginner) being separated by a large gap in experience. *Source:* Based on Dreyfus and Dreyfus (1980).

decisions that they often silently make while they perform the skill. Why does a teacher stand where they stand? What are they looking for in that moment? What are they feeling for? Is there a sound they are using to tell them something? How do they know it is safe to proceed with the procedure after taking a time-out? All of these things are very important to novice learners, but teachers may not always tell them what they are thinking because they are not even thinking about it – performing the procedure is automatic and they "just know how to do it." Students should feel comfortable asking their teachers to stop and tell them why, without being made to feel bad about asking! Students are there to learn and it can be very formative to have a student ask a teacher to reflect on how they came to do things a certain way.

Despite all this, experts sometimes disagree on the steps involved to achieve a skill, and while they may be able to come to a general consensus on how to teach it to novice learners, there may be times where they agree to disagree and the student is left to assimilate two different ways of doing something when all they want is to be shown THE way (Sullivan et al., 2014; Wingfield et al., 2015). Students should be open to, and accepting of, this type of situation and appreciate that there is always going to be more than one way of doing the same thing and that they will eventually settle on their own way of doing it after they learn what works for them.

Conclusions

Evidence-based teaching methods have been developed and adopted for clinical skills teaching in veterinary medicine and have been shown to improve the performance of novice students. Expert clinicians can become more effective teachers by learning a few student-centered techniques and putting them into routine practice. The days of "see one, do one, teach one" are over and the science of learning can be harnessed to more effectively train the next generation of veterinary students.

References

Barbe, W. B., Milone, M. N. 1981. What we know about modality strengths. *Educ Leadersh.* Association for Supervision and Curriculum Development, 38, 378–380.

Bloom, B. S. (ed.). 1956. *Taxonomy of Educational Objectives, Handbook I: The Cognitive Domain.* New York: David McKay Co. Inc.

El Boghdady, M., Ewalds-Kvist, B. M. 2020. The influence of music on the surgical task performance: A systematic review. *Int J Surg,* 73, 101–112.

Bristol Veterinary School. 2017. Bristol Veterinary School Clinical Skills Booklets. http://www.bristol.ac.uk/vetscience/research/comparative-clinical/veterinary-education/clinical-skills-booklets/sutures/ Accessed February 21, 2021.

Campbell, J., Tirapelle, L., Yates, K., et al. 2011. The effectiveness of a cognitive task analysis informed curriculum to increase self-efficacy and improve performance for an open cricothyrotomy. *J Surg Educ,* 68, 403–407.

Decloedt, A., Franco, D., Martlé, V., et al. 2020. Development of surgical competence in veterinary students using a flipped classroom approach. *J Vet Med Educ*, e20190060. doi: 10.3138/jvme.2019-0060.

Dent, J. A., Hesketh, E. A. 2004. Developing the teaching instinct, 13: How to teach in the clinical skills centre. *Med Teach*, 26, 207–210.

Dilly, M., Read, E. K., Baillie, S. 2017. A survey of established veterinary clinical skills laboratories from Europe and North America: Present practices and recent developments. *J Vet Med Educ*, 44, 580–589.

Dreyfus, S. E., Dreyfus, H. L. 1980. *A Five-Stage Model of the Mental Activities Involved in Directed Skill Acquisition*. Washington, DC: Storming Media.

Dreyfus, S. E. 2004. The five stage model of adult skill acquisition. *Bull Sci Technol Soc*, 24, 177.

Edmunds, S., Brown, G. 2010. Effective small group learning: AMEE guide no. 48. *Med Teach*, 32, 715–726.

Ericsson, K. A. 2004. Deliberate practice and the acquisition and maintenance of expert performance in medicine and related domains. *Acad Med*, 79, S70–S81.

Fleming, N. D. 1995. I'm different; not dumb. Modes of presentation (VARK) in the tertiary classroom. In: Proceedings of the 1995 Annual Conference of the Higher Education and Research Development Society of Australasia, Vol. 18. Zelmer, A. (ed.), Research and development in higher education, pp. 308–313.

Frendo Londgren, M., Baillie, S. Roberts, J., et al. 2020. A survey to establish the extent of flipped classroom use prior to clinical skills laboratory teaching and determine potential benefits, challenges and possibilities. *J Vet Med Educ*, e20190137. doi: 10.3138/jvme-2019-0137.

George, J. H., Doto, F. X. 2001. A simple five-step method for teaching clinical skills. *Fam Med*, 33, 577–578.

Halsted, W. S. 1904. The training of the surgeon. *Bull Johns Hopkins Hosp*, 15, 267–275.

Irby, D. M., Papadakis, M. 2001. Does good clinical teaching really make a difference? *Am J Med*, 110, 231–232.

Irby, D. M., Bowen, J. L. 2004. Time-efficient strategies for learning and performance. *Clin Teach*, 1, 23–28.

Issenberg, S. B., McGaghie, W. C., Petrusa, E. R., et al. 2005. Features and uses of high-fidelity medical simulations that lead to effective learning: A BEME systematic review. *Med Teach*, 27, 10–28.

Johnson, S., Healey, A., Evans, J., et al. 2006. Physical and cognitive task analysis in interventional radiology. *Clin Radiol*, 61, 97–103.

Kahneman, D. 2011. *Thinking Fast and Slow*. New York, NY: Farrar, Strauss and Giroux.

Kalyuga, S., Sweller, J. 2018. Cognitive load and expertise reversal. In: *Cambridge Handbooks in Psychology. The Cambridge Handbook of Expertise and Expert Performance*. Ericsson, K. A., Hoffman, R. R., Kozbelt, A., et al. (eds.) Cambridge, UK: Cambridge University Press, pp. 793–811.

Kneebone, R. L. 2009. An approach for simulation-based surgical and procedure training. *JAMA*, 302, 1336–1338.

Kurtz, S. M., Silverman, J. D., Draper, J. 1998. *Teaching and Learning Communication Skills in Medicine*. Oxford, UK: Radcliffe Medical Press (Oxford).

Langenbæk, R., Eika, B., Jensen, A. L., et al. 2012. Anxiety in veterinary surgical students: A quantitative study. *J Vet Med Educ*, 39, 331–340.

Low-Beer, N., Kinnison, T., Baillie, S., et al. 2011. Hidden practice revealed: Using task analysis and novel simulator design to evaluate the teaching of digital rectal examination. *Am J Surg*, 201, 46–53.

Luhoway, J. A., Ryan, J. F., Istl, A. C., et al. 2019. Perceived barriers to the development of technical skill proficiency in surgical clerkship. *J Surg Educ*, 76, 1267–1277.

Luker, K. R., Sullivan, M. E., Peyre, S. E., et al. 2008. The use of a cognitive task analysis-based multimedia program to teach surgical decision making in flexor tendon repair. *Am J Surg*, 195, 11–15.

Malone, E. 2019. Challenges & issues: Evidence-based clinical skills teaching and learning: What do we really know? *J Vet Med Educ*, 46, 379–398.

Matthew, S. M., Schoenfeld-Tacher, R. M., Danielson, J. A., et al. 2019. Flipped classroom use in veterinary education: A multinational survey of faculty experiences. *J Vet Med Educ*, 46, 97–107.

McGaghie, W. C., Issenberg S. B., Petrusa, E. R., et al. 2010. A critical review of simulation-based medical education research: 2003–2009. *Med Educ*, 44, 50–63.

McGaghie, W. C., Issenberg, S. B., Cohen, E. R., et al. 2011. Does simulation-based medical education with deliberate practice yield better results than traditional clinical education? A meta-analytic comparative review of the evidence. *Acad Med*, 86, 706–711.

Miller, G. E. 1990. The assessment of clinical skills/competence/performance. *Acad Med*, 65, s63–s67.

Moffett, J. 2015. Twelve tips for "flipping" the classroom. *Med Teach*, 37, 331–336.

Molloy, E., Boud, D. 2013. Seeking a different angle on feedback in clinical education: the learner as seeker, judge and user of performance information. *Med Educ*, 47, 227–229.

Morin, D. E., Arnold, C. J., Hale-Mitchell, L. K., et al. 2020. Development and evolution of the clinical skills learning center as an integral component of the Illinois veterinary professional curriculum. *J Vet Med Educ*, 47, 307–320.

Moulton, C., Regehr, G., Lingard, L., et al. 2010. Slowing down to stay out of trouble in the operating room: Remaining attentive in automaticity. *Acad Med*, 85, 1571–1577.

Müller, L. R., Tipold, A., Ehlers, J. P., et al. 2019. TiHoVideos: Veterinary students' utilization of instructional videos on clinical skills. *BMC Vet Res*, 15, 326–337.

Neher, J. O., Gordon, K. C., Meyer, B., et al. 1992. A five-step "microskills" model of clinical teaching. *J Am Board Fam Pract*, 5, 419–424.

Newman, L. R., Roberts, D. H., Frankl, S. E. 2019. Twelve tips for providing feedback to peers about their teaching. *Med Teach*, 41, 1118–1123.

Norman, G. R., Grierson, L. E. M., Sherbino, J., et al. 2018. Expertise in medicine and surgery. In: *Cambridge Handbooks in Psychology. The Cambridge Handbook of Expertise and Expert Performance*. Ericsson, K. A., Hoffman, R. R., Kozbelt, A., et al. (eds.) Cambridge, UK: Cambridge University Press, pp. 331–355.

Ramani, S., Leinster, S. 2008. AMEE guide no. 34: Teaching in the clinical environment. *Med Teach*, 30, 347–364.

Read, E. K., Baillie, S. 2013. Using cognitive task analysis (CTA) to create a teaching protocol for bovine dystocia. *J Vet Med Educ*, 40, 397–401.

Read, E. K., Hecker, K. G. 2013. The development and delivery of a systematic veterinary clinical skills education program at the University of Calgary. *Vet Sci Technol*, S4. doi: 10.4172/2157-7579.S4-004.

Read, E., Vallevand, A., Farrell, R. 2016. Evaluation of veterinary student surgical skills preparation for ovariohysterectomy using simulators: A pilot study. *J Vet Med Educ*, 42, 190–213.

Scalese, R. J., Issenberg, S. B. 2005. Effective use of simulations for the teaching and acquisition of veterinary professional and clinical skills. *J Vet Med Educ*, 32, 461–467.

Siddiqui, Z. S., Jonas-Dwyer, D., Carr, S. E. 2007. Twelve tips for peer observation of teaching. *Med Teach*, 29, 297–300.

Smeak, D. D. 2007. Teaching surgery to the veterinary novice: the Ohio State University experience. *J Vet Med Educ*, 34, 620–627.

Smink, D. S., Peyre, S. E., Soybel, D. I., et al. 2012. Utilization of a cognitive task analysis for laparoscopic appendectomy to identify differentiated intraoperative teaching objectives. *Am J Surg*, 203, 540–545.

Smith, D. T., Kohlwes, R. J. 2011. Teaching strategies used by internal medicine residents on the wards. *Med Teach*, 33, e697–e703.

Sullivan, M. E., Brown, C. V. R., Peyre, S. E., et al. 2007. The use of cognitive task analysis to improve the learning of percutaneous tracheostomy placement. *Am J Surg*, 193, 96–99.

Sullivan, M. E., Ortega, A., Wasserberg, N., et al. 2008. Assessing the teaching of procedural skills: Can cognitive task analysis add to our traditional teaching methods? *Am J Surg*, 195, 20–23.

Sullivan, M. E., Yates, K. A., Inaba, K., et al. 2014. The use of cognitive task analysis to reveal the instructional limitations of experts in the teaching of procedural skills. *Acad Med*, 89, 1–6.

Tomorrow's Doctors. 2009. Authorship Credit is the General Medical Council. https://www.kcl.ac. uk/lsm/study/outreach/downloads/tomorrows-doctors.pdf Accessed: February 21, 2021.

Vanka, A., Hovaguimian, A. 2019. Teaching strategies for the clinical environment. *Clin Teach*, 16, 570–574.

Velmahos, G. C., Toutouzas, K. G., Sillin, L. F., et al. 2004. Cognitive task analysis for teaching technical skills in an inanimate surgical skills laboratory. *Am J Surg*, 187, 114–119.

Walker, M., Peyton, J. 1998. *Teaching in Theatre. Teaching and Learning in Medical Practice.* Rickmansworth, UK: Manticore Europe Limited, pp. 171–180.

Warman, S. M., Pritchard, J., Baillie, S. 2015. Faculty development for a new curriculum: Implementing a strategy for veterinary teachers within the wider university context. *J Vet Med Educ*, 42, 1–7. doi: 10.3138/ jvme.1214-124R1.

Wingfield, L. R., Kulendran, M., Chow, A., et al. 2015. Cognitive task analysis: Bringing olympic athlete style training to surgical education. *Surg. Innov.*, 22, 406–417.

Yates, K., Sullivan, M., Clark, R. 2012. Integrated studies on the use of cognitive task analysis to capture surgical expertise for central venous catheter placement and open cricothyrotomy. *Am J Surg*, 203, 76–80.

Young, J. Q., Van Merrienboer, J., Durning, S., et al. 2014. Cognitive load theory: Implications for medical education: AMEE guide no. 86. *Med Teach*, 36, 371–384.

4

How Are Clinical Skills Practiced?

Emma K. Read[1] and Robin Farrell[2]

[1] College of Veterinary Medicine, The Ohio State University, Columbus, OH, USA
[2] UCD School of Veterinary Medicine, University College Dublin, Dublin, Ireland

---

Box 4.1   Key Messages

- Individuals require varied amounts of practice to acquire clinical skills proficiency
- Learning curves can be useful to track progress and help predict the amount of practice required to achieve competence.
- Attaining competence in one skill affects learning for other skills
- Deliberate practice and receiving specific feedback are key factors in the acquisition and maintenance of clinical skills proficiency

- Regular reflection can aid in identifying clinical skills that may need more or less practice
- Without regular practice individuals will experience a forgetting curve and skill proficiency will decline
- Procedural and contextual knowledge are critical components of clinical skills training that must be emphasized in practice situations
- A clinical skills laboratory is a useful location to engage in practice of psychomotor skills

---

Introduction

Learning a new skill can be daunting, but there are several key factors that can enhance learning and ease the process of both acquiring, and maintaining, clinical skills. Veterinary clinical skills vary widely in their complexity across a range of species and, when combined together, several individual skills can be incorporated into a procedure. Skills are often taught in controlled settings such as practice laboratories or skills centers where students can focus on either a single skill or a cluster of skills at one time. The controlled setting means that students are encouraged to break skills down into their component parts as they are learning, with time spent revisiting the parts that are causing them more difficulty over and over until they are mastered.

In the clinic or workplace, it is often impossible to dissociate various skills from one another to allow specific practice of any one component. As well, there is often little time for assessment, making it more challenging for students to grasp the component parts of procedures (Elder, 2018). *In situ* practice also does not typically allow the same skill to be

Veterinary Clinical Skills, First Edition. Edited by Emma K. Read, Matt R. Read, and Sarah Baillie.
© 2022 John Wiley & Sons, Inc. Published 2022 by John Wiley & Sons, Inc.
Companion website: www.wiley.com/go/read/veterinary

practiced over and over in a short period of time, with gradual escalation of difficulty, continuous self-reflection, and low-stakes risk to patients and clients (Mitchell and Boyer, 2020).

Clinical skills laboratories were first used in medicine to help train medical students prior to their first contact with patients. As hospital caseloads increased and ethical questions were raised about using patients as learning tools, there was a shift toward simulation and creation of teaching spaces off the ward. Modern veterinary clinical skills training centers have followed suit and have been in use over the past 25 years, focusing on student-centered teaching and support (Read and Hecker, 2013; Dilly et al., 2017). These safe spaces offer the opportunity for learners to practice in a stress-free setting without fear of harming animals, and they also frequently utilize simulators and task trainers that are critical to meeting the ethical needs of the general public. In a skills training facility, students can practice repeatedly, receive regular feedback, and supplement their learning with additional resources supplied by the program (Dilly et al., 2017).

Clinical skills laboratories generally contain a variety of low fidelity models, with some also featuring high fidelity ones that are commercially available (Dilly et al., 2017). Equipment and learning resources, including videos, information and instruction booklets, and other technology pieces are also commonly made available. The amount of equipment and furniture in the actual laboratory will depend on the institution and whether the setting is purpose-built or repurposed from a former space that already contains features. Each laboratory setting is unique and built to serve the purposes of that institution and its teaching mission. Safety is an important aspect of setting up practice laboratories for learners, who are typically asked to abide by "house rules" to avoid inappropriate use of potentially dangerous chemicals, equipment, or clinical samples (Booth and Coombes, 2015). Most laboratories feature some form of restricted access for learners and only grant privileges after an orientation featuring some safety training. Initially, many clinical skills laboratories were used by students on a self-serve basis for practice with little staff to oversee their operation, but now many are being used to deliver classes as well.

As pointed out in Chapter 3, gaining competence in individual clinical skills requires students to assimilate factual knowledge (e.g. basic knowledge such as anatomy), conditional knowledge (e.g. information about patient context such as *when* to use a skill and *why* it would be helpful), and procedural knowledge (e.g. the sequence that the steps of a psychomotor skill need to be performed in), as well as learn the mechanical aspects of performing the skill itself (Michels et al., 2012). Although knowledge can be gained through reading and watching videos, gaining proficiency in psychomotor skills requires actual hands-on practice where knowledge steps are practiced and integrated with the physical activity of "doing." Knowledge learned in the context of "doing" is more easily retained and more readily processed into long-term memory (Korwin and Jones, 1990).

Clinical skills have outcomes that are amenable to objective measurement. This means instructors have the ability to assess development and mastery, and the student can be provided with specific feedback about their performance, further driving improvement (Ericsson et al., 2018). Feedback informs a student's deliberate practice, which is a process that involves exposure to skills of graded difficulty while simultaneously receiving immediate information regarding performance and, hopefully, suggestions for improvement. Research suggests that regular expert feedback, as well as the success or failure of a surgical procedure itself, is critical for development of expertise in novice surgeons (Ericsson, 2011).

In this chapter we will explore:

- how skills learning takes place and how students can best facilitate their own practice sessions;
- what types of "practice" exist and how to incorporate evidence-based methods into learning;
- how students can individualize their learning and optimize improvement through the use of learning curves; and
- how peers can help each other practice.

Practice Makes Perfect but Not All Practice Is Perfect – How a Student Ensures That They Are Learning and Practicing the Correct Method

Consider the following quotes:

> Practice does not make perfect. Only perfect practice makes perfect.
> *Vince Lombardi*
> Practice makes perfect? Practicing the wrong things over and over again, makes you even better at what you're not good at.
> *Paul Strikwerda*

Repetitive practice of any psychomotor skill is considered key to improving, as practice is the only way that you can gain the muscle memory to perform the skill with limited conscious thought. Being able to practice at an "automated" level is one goal of developing expertise (Moulton et al., 2007). Procedural learning is slower than knowledge-based declarative learning and requires many more repetitions (Ward and Zollo, 2017; Malone, 2019).

There are a number of ways to practice performing a clinical skill, but not all types of practice have equal value and practicing a skill using poor technique can lead to mastering a skill without all of the necessary steps or performing its steps in the incorrect sequence. In other words, the student becomes really good at doing the wrong thing. Poorly learned procedural skills can also seriously harm a patient. In this section of the chapter, we will focus on key elements that can enhance student practice sessions and facilitate positive productive learning sessions.

Cognitive Processes and Preparation for Practice

The Dreyfus and Dreyfus (1988) model has been used in several disciplines to describe the levels of learning during skills instruction, from learning to drive a car to performing a surgical procedure. The model describes five phases of skill development that lead from novice to expert. This model reminds us that when learning clinical skills, novices require rigid adherence to rules and tend to prefer single correct answers (Dreyfus and Dreyfus, 1988). The most foundational step in learning clinical skills is described as acquiring basic background knowledge about *why* a skill is required, *when* to use it, and *how* to properly perform it. For example, a student needs to be able to describe the procedural steps of a skill prior to attempting it for the first time, but other knowledge that goes along with the skill can be gained before or after learning the psychomotor steps. You may ask - 'Why is this?'

When first attempting a simple skill there is a significant cognitive load associated with learning the steps and translating those steps into physical activity. Recall that cognitive load theory, introduced in Chapter 3, states that a person can only process a certain amount of information at one time. The size of the human working memory means that it is easily overloaded if presented with too much new information all at once or, if problems become too complex, too soon (Kahneman, 2011; May, 2017). Once information enters the long-term memory, it is consolidated into larger blocks of information so that future retrieval and use of the information requires less working memory. "Chunking" information in the working memory will ensure it is memorized in aggregate form rather than as single facts, making recall easier (May, 2017). Therefore, consolidating the knowledge required prior to attempting the skill will reduce the student's cognitive load while learning the hands-on details and will allow more of their attention to be focused on the task at hand (Malone, 2019). The recent COVID-19 pandemic has helped to reinforce this critical understanding. The pandemic has necessitated that many clinical skills teachers make use of a "flipped classroom" model that helps prepare students for reduced hands-on time in the practice laboratory (Londgren et al., 2020). Students have been shown to better focus their attention on practicing their clinical skills if they can complete the initial steps of the cognitive learning before attending the practice session (Londgren et al., 2020). So just as we know that preparation is one of the most important contributors for success in *teaching* clinical skills, we have seen evidence firsthand that preparation is a vital consideration for *learning* as well.

As introduced in Chapter 3, George and Doto's model for teaching clinical skills lays out five steps, with the first few steps related to understanding the significance of the skill and memorizing all the appropriate steps in proper sequence (George and Doto, 2001). This learning model has been widely used and applied across health professions programs and is particularly useful for when a learner is struggling because it reduces their cognitive load (Booth and Coombes, 2015). This model is useful to students because it emphasizes different "channels" of input during the learning process (e.g. auditory, visual) and reminds us that input on more than one "channel" at the same time can prevent adequate processing of information and storage into long-term memory (Kahneman, 2011). The same focus should be used while a student practices, first asking themselves why the skill is important and when it will be used, then verbalizing "out loud" the steps required, then performing the steps, and finally seeking feedback on their performance from an instructor or peer before refining the process and starting over again.

A similar framework was also described by Walker and Peyton (1998) and included the following steps: (i) instructor demonstrating at normal speed without commentary, (ii) instructor repeating the skills demonstration but with describing all of the steps, (iii) student explaining the steps with instructor doing what the student is describing, and (iv) student performing the skill on their own (Herrmann-Werner et al., 2013). More on this framework will be covered in Chapter 8, but it is briefly mentioned here to highlight that there are numerous evidence-based methods of teaching and learning clinical skills that all aim to minimize cognitive load during learning by allowing students to acquire cognitive elements along different channels sequentially, before then assimilating this knowledge with the hands-on skill performance. A student can improve the process of learning clinical skills by focusing on the knowledge required and learning the sequence of steps before they come to the skills lab for hands-on practice (Herrmann-Werner et al., 2013).

How Should Practice Be Scheduled to Be Helpful?

When a student begins to learn hands-on skills and *how often* these sessions feature in the program are often debated among clinical teachers. The stage of learning, complexity of the task, and the training environment available may also play a role in how much and how often practice is needed (Malone, 2019). Working in small groups in a relaxed atmosphere has been shown to be highly conducive to skills learning, and utilizing peer-led classes and drop-in sessions can help support ongoing practice efforts (Dilly and Baillie, 2017).

Learning motor skills is considered most efficient when it is conducted in the shortest amount of practice time, with the longest intervals between sessions without losing skills in between (Yamada et al., 2019). There have been attempts to determine what the optimal practice session length is and what the ideal interval should be, but results to date are not definitive (Yamada et al., 2019). Essentially, there are two schools of thought regarding scheduling – either practicing a single skill repetitively on the same model or species in a block pattern before moving on to the next skill or learning in a more randomized pattern where a learner works on several skills simultaneously in short succession (Shea and Morgan, 1979).

Skills learned in a block of repetitive practice on the same model or exercise seem to lead to the quicker immediate achievement in skill compared to a more randomized pattern of learning. However, randomized practice has been shown to offer better sustained and improved performance in retention tests administered 10 days later (Shea and Morgan, 1979). No specific research has been conducted in veterinary medicine to compare the two methods to date, and scheduling of practice sessions is often done in consideration of other activities that have to be accommodated in the program or the skills center (Malone, 2019).

In health professions skills training, it may not be that one practice interval type outperforms another, but that both are necessary to allow for quick learning and long-term retention. Many medical schools are now using distributive (spaced) practice where the same skills are taught on a recurring basis rather than repetitively in large dedicated blocks of time or long laboratory sessions (Malone, 2019). Further research is needed in veterinary clinical skills to determine optimum spacing and structure of practice sessions, but extrapolation from other professions suggests that no matter the interval, regular practice and frequent reassessment of skills is essential to long-term retention and improved performance (Malone, 2019).

Recent studies in medicine have focused on learning curves to provide objective data regarding student development and the amount of repetition required (Pusic et al., 2015). With current emphasis on outcomes-based education, individualized learning plans with specific observation and assessment are highly desired and may be more useful (Norcini et al., 2018). More information on learning curves and their use is provided later in this chapter.

Deliberate Practice and Taking Time to Learn Properly

One of the key concepts that contributes to skills acquisition in other disciplines such as sports and music has been found to transfer to clinical skills training in the health care professions as well and is becoming widely emphasized. This is the theory of "deliberate practice," which was developed by the late K. Anders Ericsson. He described the elements of deliberate practice as: (i) provision of clearly defined learning objectives for specific tasks; (ii) precise, measurable metrics of performance; (iii) focused, repetitive practice of skills; and (iv) real-time, constructive, actionable, and specific feedback (Ericsson, 2004; Ericsson, 2008). Further popularized by author Malcolm Gladwell, the theory of deliberate practice became known as the "10,000-hour rule" because of Gladwell's understanding that professional sports athletes and master chess players spent this minimum period of time honing their skills before being considered at the top of their game (Gladwell, 2008).

The key to deliberate practice is that learners identify and focus on areas of deficit, with intention to seek incremental improvement that can be documented and built upon (Oermann, 2011; Compton et al., 2017). Feedback can be provided by instructors informally during practice sessions, after review of recorded sequences, or during formal high-stakes assessments (Dilly and Baillie, 2017). Ideally, students would take advantage of the resources provided to them, so they never practice or learn without somebody knowledgeable who can observe and offer insights on their performance at regular intervals. Repeating a skill incorrectly over and again can make a learner feel very confident and appear very efficient, but as those quoted at the outset of this section point out, it is easy to become good at doing the wrong things. Being confident in the wrong thing won't inspire much confidence in clients and can also be life threatening or otherwise harmful to patients. It is critical that learners get it right, not just for the sake of immediate assessment, but for their long-term performance in practice.

Deliberate practice not only gets a student started on the right track with learning skills properly but also ensures that they keep their skills well-honed. Practice aligned with constructive coaching that provides immediate feedback on skills performance has also been shown to be essential to slow down the decay of acquired skills (Moulton et al., 2006; Reznick and MacRae, 2006). More on this will be covered in the discussion of "forgetting curves" later in this chapter.

Reflective Practice and Working on Steady Improvement

If health professionals see knowledge or skills attainment as a finite end goal unto itself, then their practice over time will not likely change that much. Ideally, a developing health professional will come to see learning as part of a cycle of continuous self-improvement where new knowledge and skills can be integrated with those already learned, ultimately leading to a change in everyday practice. In other words, one's goal should be of constantly learning and improving one's effectiveness, not simply learning how to perform a new skill. Health professions educators refer to this as "lifelong learning" and believe that continual evolution of one's practice is not only critical to those we serve but also critical to practitioner well-being by helping to provide personal contentment with one's role in the profession (de Groot and Mastenbroek, 2017). Boyd and Fales (1983) and Boud et al. (1985) describe self-awareness and learning from one's own experiences as central to effective reflective practice. Reflective practice has been described in veterinary medicine and has documented that learners are able to look back on, learn from, and improve upon their own performance (Mastenbroek et al., 2015). Also, the recently defined competency-based veterinary education (CBVE) framework emphasizes self-directed learning as an important competency for graduates to keep honing their skills over the lifetime of their career as new techniques, knowledge, and equipment are introduced (Molgaard et al., 2018).

Reflective practice has been defined as "reflection-*on*-action" and "reflection-*in*-action," with both being important for clinical skills performance (de Groot and Mastenbroek, 2017). Reflection-*on*-action refers to the ability of a learner to look back at their past performance and make useful changes. This is likely what most novices think of when first hearing about reflective practice. Useful methods of capturing evidence of performance include video recordings, as well as verbal or written observations by experts and trained peers. A veterinarian who places a cast on a horse that the horse then subsequently breaks might reflect on whether there was a fault in the method of application that lead to weakness of the initial structure. Making changes based on lessons learned is reflection-*on*-action.

Compare this with reflection-*in*-action, which emphasizes that a veterinarian must have enough background knowledge to apply it in the moment and adapt their skills as needed to fit a specific patient's needs. A veterinarian applying a cast to a horse must decide whether to construct the cast differently when evaluating the environment that the horse lives in, as well as the client's willingness to follow care instructions. The ability to "make changes on the fly" is reflection-*in*-action. Both types of reflective practice are critical for the veterinarian to adapt their skills to the context of a patient and/or client and to react positively to learning experiences presented in everyday practice life.

It is important for veterinary students to not only develop reflective practice as an important skill for lifelong learning that they will need later in the workplace but to also learn the principles of how to apply this method in the practice laboratory as they are learning new skills. Reflecting on *what* they are doing, *why* they are doing what they are doing, and *how* they might ultimately achieve a higher level of performance is part of critical reflection during learning. The student also needs to develop resilience in learning so that when mistakes are made or tough feedback is received, the student can see this as part of the larger context where the expert instructor is trying to help the student progress in their skills development. Feedback, while personalized, is not personal and should be reflected upon as an opportunity for improvement (Stone and Heen, 2014).

Mindfulness Practice and Focusing on the Task at Hand

Mindfulness is described as the ability to be aware of and accept the present-moment experience that is happening, combined with being able to put attention where it needs to be put for the given task at hand. Mindfulness-based intervention (MBI) has been shown to improve sports-based performance as well as decrease performance-based anxiety (Rothlin et al., 2016; Buhlmayer et al., 2017). Mindfulness in veterinary students has been shown to decrease stress levels and increase their sense of calm immediately prior to operating on live patients (Stevens et al., 2019). Students performing surgery for the first time were reportedly in the 90th–95th percentile of salivary cortisol measures for general public in the same age range. Those who had undergone MBI demonstrated significant reduction in salivary cortisol levels and in self-reported stress and anxiety. Practicing mindfulness may soon be a useful part of skills training curricula and a valuable way to improve resiliency for students.

Growth Mindset

An important part of being mindful is maintaining a *growth mindset*. Researched and described extensively by Dweck (2007), a growth mindset occurs when an individual thrives on challenge and interprets it as an opportunity for stretching their existing ability. In this way, growth is a continually moving target. Compare this with a *fixed mindset* where intelligence and ability are considered innate capabilities that can't be meaningfully changed. Avoiding failure at all costs then becomes imperative, and the student seeks to avoid assessment where the learner interprets the results to mean that they don't measure up and never will (Dweck, 2007). Many veterinary students tend to be overachievers, demonstrating from a young age a keen sense of ambition and perfectionism (Kogan et al., 2020). The very traits that help them to outcompete others to enter veterinary school might later hamper their efforts to reach their full potential as they actively work to avoid failure or embarrassment. "Impostor syndrome" is a well-known challenge for many veterinary learners, and perfectionism can often exacerbate the condition because these individuals tend to be harsher critics of themselves once they fail to live up to their own exacting standards (Hamood, 2020). A recent study of international veterinarians determined that 68% of those responding met the threshold for declaration of intense imposter feelings, with younger female practitioners being at the greatest risk (Kogan et al., 2020).

Given the intensity of this issue, it is critical for instructors to emphasize a growth mindset during veterinary training and for students to consider feedback to be a gift that others offer with the goal of improving their performance. A closer look at learning curves in the next section of this chapter might help to convince skeptical readers that everyone starts out at differing points on the common learning journey and that we all have ownership of where we peak in our abilities, not because we are born with certain gifts, but because we learn how to learn and put the time in to practice while responding to the feedback from others. For more information on growth mindset, the reader is referred to Chapter 6.

Box 4.2   Practice Makes Perfect – How to Improve Your Skills for a Lifetime

- Use evidence-based teaching and learning models to help guide practice and learning sessions. This will help minimize cognitive overload
- Work on improving the "little things" – watch for details that differentiate techniques or procedures
- Alternate between block and randomized patterns of learning to maximize efficiency and retention of skills
- Seek specific feedback from observers to know where and how to improve. Accept feedback as a "gift" from others that is aimed at helping you achieve your goals more quickly
- Have a sense of humor about your mistakes and be patient with yourself

- Put in the time (remember the 10,000-hour rule). Seize every opportunity to work on making your skills better and don't stop doing so when you complete your training. Practice is a lifelong commitment
- Reflect – *on-* and *in*-practice. Always look for opportunities to improve. Be open to change and make adaptations "on the fly" wherever necessary to modify your skills to fit the situation at hand
- Be mindful – focus your attention on the task and use assessment as an opportunity to grow
- Maintain a *growth mindset* – learning is intended to be a challenge and an opportunity to stretch your skills. Take advantage of that every day

Learning Curves and Their Implications for Clinical Skills Practice

What Are Learning Curves and What Are They Used for?

Learning curves were originally used in industry to describe production gains as changes were made to manufacturing processes. Learning curves were minimally used in health professions education prior to 2001 with only 10 articles being published before that time that focused mostly on uptake of new surgical skills for minimally invasive surgery (Valsamis et al., 2018). Now, more than 200 articles have been published and collectively they inform research, education, training program development, and assessment of performance (Valsamis et al., 2018).

Learning curves in the medical education literature are essentially the graphical relationship between learning effort and achievement of performance (Howard et al., 2020). These curves can be used to describe, explain, and predict learning and show the difference in *rate* of learning due to a specific intervention (e.g. practicing with a particular model) (Howard et al., 2020). Although learning curves may vary in their shape, research suggests that acquisition of skills generally follows a similar and recognizable shape – a rapid start, followed by a progressively diminishing learning rate, and culminating in a plateau. Complex tasks also feature a period of unlearning where learners "dip down" or regress in skill before being able to "tune up" their performance again. This is called the "forgetting curve" (Pusic et al., 2017).

A typical learning curve has the following features (see Figure 4.1):

- Units of repetition (or effort) are placed on the x-axis (e.g. number of attempts).
- Outcome/performance variable is placed on the y-axis (e.g. increments of improvement).
- A y-intercept shows the learner's baseline skill level (learners rarely ever have no experience at all).

- A nonlinear slope reflects learning efficiency in terms of performance improvement with practice (i.e. rate of learning).
- An inflection point is present where the slope flattens out and increasingly greater effort is required for continued performance improvement. Learning becomes much more difficult from this point.
- An asymptote (the point at which the curve truly flattens out) is the theoretical maximum performance in the system (the so-called expert performance level).

Learning curves can be used to track progress for individual students performing individual skills or procedures where multiple skills are performed together. Recent studies have shown that not only can we track an individual student's learning curves over time but we can also track an progress for a whole cohort of students as well (Bok et al., 2018; Read et al., 2020). Learning curves can provide students with information about their own individual development, while also allowing them to compare their position relative to other learners in a group. Learning curves can help teachers to see how quickly students are progressing individually and collectively, as well as allow for an estimate where students are, or will be, in the learning process (Howard et al., 2020). Ultimately, learning curves can be used to compare cohorts of students across institutions, and this desire among educators has led to development of common frameworks for learning (Matthew et al., 2020). More on this will be discussed in the section on outcomes-based education at the end of the chapter.

How Are Learning Curves Used in Clinical Skills Education?

Learning curves (e.g. with respect to acquiring psychomotor skills) can vary considerably for each individual learner but follow the same typical pattern of gradual increase in development over time before leveling off at the competent or proficient level. There is limited research to date in the area of learning curves specific to veterinary clinical skills. One study

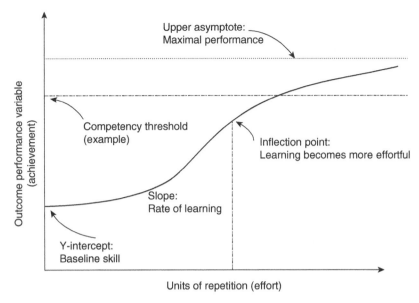

Figure 4.1 A generic representation of the learning curve demonstrating key concepts in the relationship between the y-axis or performance, and the x-axis or effort. Adapted from Howard et al., 2020.

included a group of veterinary students with no previous experience who attempted to place an intravenous catheter in a partial training simulator (Campbell et al., 2014). In that study, there was a large variability reported in the speed at which they became proficient in catheter placement – one student was able to attain proficiency in placing an intravenous catheter after attempting it only 18 times while another student required 55 attempts to reach the end goal. Other students repeated the task more than 60 times and had not yet become proficient by the end of the study. This work also informed where learners had trouble with different aspects of the task, and tracking performance of all the steps to completion allowed instructors to tailor individualized feedback for correction of errors more rapidly than for learners who did not receive such feedback.

The shape of an individual's learning curve tells a lot about their journey toward competence. Did the student start out quickly and then stall in terms of mastering the more complicated aspects of the task or procedure? Was the student simply not as advanced as others at the baseline and then struggled to keep up?

Learning curves can be a basis for conversation with instructors about how best to improve their teaching and where difficulties are arising with their students. Learning curves can also be useful to learners by helping them to become self-regulated. They can show their past performance and plot out their anticipated progress, which will motivate them to work through challenges to attain a higher level of skill without losing interest in repetitive practice. Ultimately, learning curves may be more meaningful feedback for self-appraisal than comparing one's self to the mean score on an Objective Structured Clinical Examination (OSCE).

Group-level analyses allow the instructor to determine from which level most learners are starting and also provide information on where the asymptote falls (i.e. the level at which the majority of learners will attain proficiency). Such analyses help the instructor determine how many repetitions may be required before learners are proficient (Bok et al., 2018).

Tracking of learners using learning curves might also allow for individuals with slower progress to be identified and provided with extra practice to catch them up. Groups of students can be targeted for additional support rather than assigning work for all students based on a set number of trials or a specific duration spent on task. Resources can be concentrated where they are required.

Do Learning Curves Essentially Look the Same?

Learning curves do not look alike from one individual or one cohort to the next, but there are a few recognizable patterns that are common:

1) "Diminishing returns curve." When the task is easy to learn, there is a period of rapid progression before learning plateaus (Figure 4.2).
2) "Increasing returns curve." When the task is hard to learn, there is a period of slow progress before the task starts to be mastered and the learning accelerates (Figure 4.3).
3) "The S curve." When a learner is really new to a task, they learn slowly at first before becoming more proficient. Learning then occurs rapidly before finally reaching a plateau, reflecting the point at which they attain mastery (Figure 4.4) (Murre, 2014).
4) "The complex curve." It is most often seen with procedural tasks in medicine. Several phases exist, and the rate of learning is variable along the length of the curve. The phases end with a period of overlearning once peak proficiency is surpassed, and there is a "forgetting curve" without continued

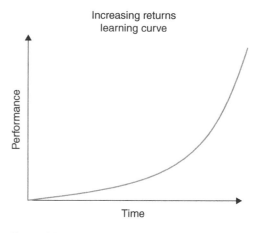

Figure 4.3   Increasing returns learning curve.

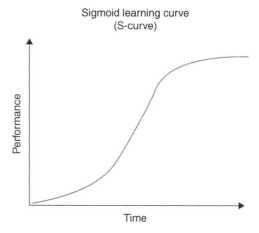

Figure 4.4   Sigmoid (S-curve) learning curve.

practice at regular intervals (more on this later in this chapter) (Figures 4.5 and 4.7) (Pusic et al., 2015).

Figures 4.2–4.7 show common learning curves (figures adapted from Valsamis et al., 2018 and Pusic et al., 2011).

Differentiating Expertise – Becoming an Automatic Versus Deliberate Expert

Research in learning curves has also informed the notion that there are differences in expertise, and this is an important concept to emphasize to students. How you practice and how much additional effort you put in once you start to plateau

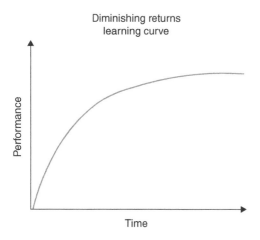

Figure 4.2   Diminishing returns learning curve.

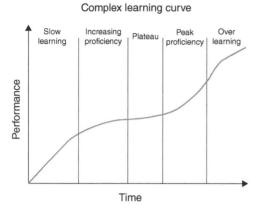

Figure 4.5 Complex learning curve.

determine if you can take your performance to an even higher level still. Once a student becomes an expert (as defined by when they reach the asymptote or when they plateau in skill attainment), their performance becomes automated (Kalet and Pusic, 2014). At this point, they can perform the skill without putting much thought into it and the physical skill can often be performed quickly and efficiently with "muscle memory." If an "automatic expert" wishes to improve beyond this level of plateau, they must put in extraordinary effort to incrementally drive their learning upward again. But it is possible. This extra effort and achievement are associated with becoming a "deliberate expert" or "adaptive expert" (Kalet and Pusic, 2014; Pusic et al., 2015). Effort is still required to be better, and the expert must look for the little things that they can tweak

or improve on in order to drive their performance to the next level. Students with fixed mindsets often never progress past being an automatic expert because they don't seek out the additional feedback and practice needed. A growth mindset will encourage the development of deliberate expertise as the student remains open to feedback and seeks new ways to push themselves to mastery. They view the end point as a "game to keep playing" rather than as a "destination to arrive at." The more complicated modern veterinary medicine becomes (and the more there is to learn in a four-year curriculum), the more emphasis there will need to be on students becoming deliberate experts (Pusic et al., 2015) (Figure 4.6).

What Are Forgetting Curves and Why Are They Important?

Incorporation of a *complex learning curve* with a *forgetting curve* has been termed an "experience curve." This can be used to describe development and learning that is typical across a wide variety of health professions career paths (Hatala et al., 2019).

Forgetting curves occur when students learn skills at nonlinear rates following a period of nonpractice. Recent research has focused on predicting when forgetting will occur for average students and at what interval practice must be maintained in order to avoid further decay (Howard et al., 2020). Making students explicitly aware that there is a "forgetting curve" can also motivate them to pursue additional training or refreshers, and knowing roughly when this is likely to occur can help schedule when remedial training should occur.

Do Students Begin at the Same Point? Consider the Y-intercept

Having talked about where students will end up on a learning curve and what they need to do to stay at the "top of their game," we need to consider that some students will have a "head start" on their peers because of where they begin. Different students who are provided the same instruction may experience it differently and may therefore learn at different rates (Hatala

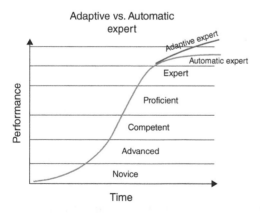

Figure 4.6 Adaptive versus automatic expert (adapted from Pusic et al. 2011).

The forgetting curve

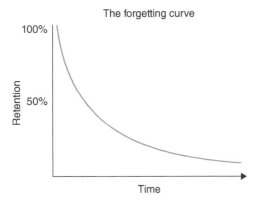

Figure 4.7 Forgetting curve.

et al., 2019). Also, students arrive with different levels of background knowledge or skill as they enter a training program (i.e. a greater y-intercept) that places them at a higher location on the learning curve before they even start learning (Pusic et al., 2015; Pusic et al., 2018).

The rate of learning can influence how a learner perceives and develops a practice schedule for clinical skills training. Initial rapid acquisition of skills can lead to a false sense of competency, whereas later slow-perfecting of skill can cause increasing frustration. Both may lead to reduced willingness to practice (Malone, 2019). Setting performance *process* goals that focus on the "how" of the skill, rather than performance *outcome* goals that focus on the "what" or "achievement" of steps in the skill, can help better motivate learners. Following development of performance process goals using a learning curve can help a learner to recognize that progress is being made in fine increments and encourage them to stick with it (Brydges et al., 2009; Malone, 2019). Learners who start out behind their peers will be encouraged to persevere until they catch up. Importantly, it is worth noting that it is the rare student who is ahead in every area. In a class of veterinary students, individuals will typically have different levels of experience, leading to a wide range of y-intercepts. Peers should be encouraged to learn from one another and to help one another, so they can capitalize on each other's prior experiences in different areas.

How Do Learning Curves Fit in with the Current Trend in Outcomes-based Education? How Does This Help Development in Clinical Practice?

In many countries, the veterinary profession features an accreditation system that defines standards that must be met by students and educational institutions (e.g. American Veterinary Medical Association Council on Education [AVMA COE] accreditation standards, Royal College of Veterinary Surgeons [RCVS] Day One competences, and Accreditation Committee for Veterinary Nurse Education [ACOVENE]). Before completing their training program, it is expected that a veterinary or veterinary nursing student will reach a certain level of competence or proficiency on a defined list of day one competencies, including clinical skills.

The recently described AAVMC's (Association of American Veterinary Medical Colleges) CBVE framework was developed to define common outcomes shared among veterinary institutions, no matter which accreditation system they use, and describes 9 domains and 32 competencies with a series of milestones for each competency whereby the learner progresses from novice to proficient (Salisbury et al., 2019; Matthew et al., 2020). The CBVE framework also incorporates eight entrustable professional activities (EPAs), which are essential tasks that learners can be trusted with, once sufficient competence has been demonstrated (Molgaard et al., 2019). These EPAs incorporate multiple competencies (i.e. skills, knowledge, values, and attitudes) into one single task or procedure that can be assessed by an experienced clinician who can then provide feedback to the learner using an entrustment scale (Salisbury et al., 2020). See Figure 4.8 for an example of an EPA that can be assessed using the accompanying entrustment scale.

Entrustment scales provide information to the learner about any of the following, depending on the particular scale used:

- how much the assessor trusts them to perform the skill in the future based on what they saw at a specific moment in time ("Prospective" – Figure 4.8),

- how much of the task they actually saw the learner do ("Retrospective" – e.g. learner required minimal supervision; could be trusted to do on own if already graduated), and
- how much they as an assessor had to assist the learner with ("Retrospective" – e.g. I had to talk them through the task).

No matter which entrustment scale is used, the goal is for the learner to receive feedback about what was observed, including what the student needs to keep doing and what improvements are needed the next time the task is attempted.

Repeated feedback and placing the student on a series of milestones along a continuum of practice development from novice to proficient can help to document the rate of their development over time (Salisbury et al., 2019). Such a graph is ultimately a learning curve and can be used to evaluate an individual's performance in the clinical workplace, as well as allow for comparison between learners – it is a snapshot evaluation of an entire cohort (Bok et al., 2018). Learning curves not only have a place in the practice lab and clinical skills teaching sessions but also have a place in monitoring progress in the practice workplace.

Making the Most of Peer Support for Practice

By this point in the chapter, it should be clear why practice is important and how to determine if progress is being made. It has also been advocated that the Clinical Skills center is the ideal place for a developing student to hone their skills because of the access to experts and instructional materials including a variety of models. Despite all the advantages offered by institutions in the skills center, there remains one very important resource that has to be sought out by the student themselves. A friend. Near-peer (close in training but not exactly the same in experience level) and peer-to-peer (same experience level) practice sessions are useful to encourage learners to attend labs and make use of the resources provided (Molgaard and Read, 2017). Some lab managers have reported that skills labs are infrequently used for practice except for the period of time immediately prior to summative assessments (Malone, 2019). As stated above, regular practice sessions with frequent feedback are more likely

Student name: "Student"	Don't trust to perform	Trust but needs a lot of help to perform	Trust but needs some help to perform	Trust to perform on own
CBVE EPA #2 - develop a diagnostic plan and interpret results		X		
What went well:	"Student" could develop a problem list and accurately identified abnormalities with the patient.			
Next time please try:	"Student" could use further reading to help strengthen their knowledge of differential diagnoses that match up with the identified problems. A better understanding of available diagnoses would also help to sort differential diagnoses by priority.			

Figure 4.8 Example of a completed EPA assessed with an entrustment scale (Read et al., 2020).

to improve and maintain skills than sporadic yet exhaustive sessions. A recent study showed two short sessions a week in a peer-directed setting were adequate to make a significant difference in skills retention and performance for students (Compton et al., 2017). Working with a peer tutor can strongly encourage use of the skills center and can provide someone from whom to offer specific feedback that can help improve performance. Peer-assisted learning is useful for formative assessment and can be especially helpful for preparing for high-stakes, summative assessment (e.g. OSCEs). Not only do tutees benefit but tutors are also forced to reflect on their own content gaps and develop a deeper understanding of the nuances of the skills they are teaching. In fact, studies have shown a higher level of performance on OSCEs for peer tutors (Knobe et al., 2010). See Chapter 8 for more information on Peer-Assisted Learning.

Conclusion

Practice is necessary for learning and improving clinical skills. Many resources exist that can be used to significant advantage for practice, but an understanding of how best to structure efforts is important to maximize benefits. A smart student seeks specific feedback, uses

---

Box 4.3 **Making the Most of the Clinical Skill Laboratory for Practice**
• Prepare ahead of time and arrive with knowledge, ready to go   • Observe safety rules and practices   • Make use of a variety of models and resources   • Seek peer support and feedback   • Attend regularly – make it a habit   • Clean up after yourself and respect your colleagues

---

evidence-based learning methods, maintains a growth mindset, and learns from their mistakes. Learning data can be useful to help determine practice repetitions necessary as well as ideal intervals between skills refreshment. Individual students and cohorts can be monitored for improvement, and struggling learners can be identified for targeted assistance. Development of expertise can be monitored, and evidence of learning can be used to fulfill accreditation requirements regarding student achievement. Students should seek to work with others as they practice their skills and be open to the feedback that others can provide. Ultimately, prepared students who enter the skills center with a plan to take advantage of all it can offer will be the ones who progress the fastest and have the most to take with them when they enter the practice workplace.

References

Bok, H. G. J., de Jong, L. H., O'Neill, T., et al. 2018. Validity evidence for programmatic assessment in competency-based education. *Perspect Med Educ*, 7, 362–372.

Booth, N., Coombes, N. 2015. Effective learning of practical clinical skills. In: *Guidebook for Developing Veterinary Clinical Skills Laboratories (CSL's)* http://creativecommons. org/licenses/by-nc-nd/4.0/ or http://www. bristol.ac.uk/media-library/sites/vetscience/ documents/clinical-skills/House%20Rules.pdf.

Boyd, E. M., Fales, A. W. 1983. Reflective learning. *J Humanis Psycho*, 23, 99–117.

Boud, D., Kehoe R., Walker, D. 1985. Promoting reflection in learning; a model. In: *Turning Experience into Learning*. Boud D., Keogh, R.,

Walker, D. (eds.) London: Croon Helm, pp. 18–40. Accessed (1.3.21) at: https://books. google.com/books?hl=en&lr=&id=MVvdAA AAQBAJ&oi=fnd&pg=PA32&dq=Boyd+D.,+ Kehoe+R.,+and+Walker+D.+(1985)+Promot ing+reflection+in+learning%3B+a+model+i n+reflectitin.+In:+Boyd+D.,+Keogh+R.,+W alker+D.,+eds.+Turning+Experience+into+ Learning.+Kogan+Page,+London:+18- 40&ots=CIfgHwKZy2&sig=eTkp3S6RECAm5 zHgfknL2DdizAk#v=onepage&q&f=false.

Brydges, R., Carnahan, H., Safir, O., et al. 2009. How effective is self-guided learning of clinical technical skills? It's all about process. *Med Educ*, 43, 507–515.

Buhlmayer, L., Birrer, D., Rothlin, P., et al. 2017. Effects of mindfulness practice on performance-relevant parameters and performance outcomes in sports: a meta-analytical review. *Sports Med*, 47, 2309–2321.

Campbell, R. D., Hecker, K. G., Biau, D. J., et al. 2014. Student attainment of proficiency in a clinical skill: The assessment of individual learning curves. *PLoS One*, 9, e88526.

Compton, N. J., Cary, J. A., Wenz, J. R., et al. 2017. Evaluation of peer teaching and deliberate practice to teach veterinary surgery. *Vet. Surg*, 48, 99–208.

de Groot E., Mastenbroek, N. J. J. M. 2017. Lifelong learning and reflective practice. In: *Veterinary Medical Education: A Practical Guide.* Hodgson, J. L., Pelzer, J. M. (eds.) Hoboken, NJ: John Wiley & Sons, Inc., pp. 433–447.

Dilly, M., Baillie, S. 2017. Learning and teaching in clinical skills laboratories. In: *Veterinary Medical Education: A Practical Guide.* Hodgson, J. L., Pelzer, J. M. (eds.) Hoboken, NJ: John Wiley & Sons, Inc., pp. 151–161.

Dilly, M., Read, E. K., Baillie, S. 2017. A survey of established veterinary clinical skills laboratories from Europe and North America: Present practices and recent developments. *J Vet Med Educ*, 44, 580–589.

Dreyfus, H. L., Dreyfus, S. E. 1988. *Mind Over Machine.* New York, NY: Free Press.

Dweck, C. 2007. *Mindset. The New Psychology of Success. How We Can Learn to Fulfil Our Potential.* New York, NY: Ballantine Books.

Ericsson, K. A. 2004. Deliberate practice and the acquisition and maintenance of expert performance in medicine and related domains. *Acad Med*, 79, S70–81.

Ericsson, K. A. 2008. Deliberate practice and acquisition of expert performance: A general overview. *Acad Emerg Med*, 15, 988–994.

Ericsson, K. A. 2011. The surgeon's expertise. In: *Surgical Education: Theorising an Emerging Domain.* Fry, H., Kneebone, R. (eds.) Dordrecht: Springer, pp.107–121.

Ericsson, K. A., Hoffman, R. R., Kozbelt, A., et al. 2018. *The Cambridge Handbook of Expertise and Expert Performance*, 2nd Edition. Anders Ericsson, K., Hoffman, R. R., Kozbelt, A. et al. (eds.) Cambridge, UK: Cambridge University Press.

Elder, A. 2018. Clinical skills assessment. *Med Clin North Am*, 102, 545–558.

Londgren, M. F., Baillie S., Roberts, J., et al. 2020. A survey to establish the extent of flipped classroom use prior to clinical skills laboratory teaching and determine potential benefits, challenges, and possibilities. *J Vet Med Educ*, e20190137.

George, J. H., Doto, F. X. 2001. A simple five-step method for teaching clinical skills. *Fam Med*, 33, 577–578.

Gladwell, M. 2008. *Outliers: The Story of Success.* New York, NY: Little, Brown and Company.

Hamood, W. 2020. Imposter syndrome and the veterinary profession. *Vet Rec*, 187, 268–270.

Hatala, R., Gutman, J., Lineberry, M., et al. 2019. How well is each learner learning? Validity investigation of a learning curve-based assessment approach for ECG interpretation. *Adv Health Sci Educ Theory Pract*, 24, 45–63.

Herrmann-Werner, A., Nikendel, C., Keifenheim, K., et al. 2013. "Best practice" skills lab training vs. a "see one, do one" approach in undergraduate medical education: An RCT on students' long-term ability to perform procedural clinical skills. *PLoS One*, 8, 1–13.

Howard, N., Cook, D., Hatala, R., et al. 2020. Learning curves in health professions education simulation research. A systematic review. *Simul Healthc*, doi: https://doi.org/10.1097/SIH.0000000000000477.

Kahneman, D. 2011. *Thinking, Fast and Slow*. Basingstoke: Macmillan.

Kalet, A., Pusic, M. 2014. Defining and assessing competence. In: *Remediation in Medical Education*, 1st Edition. Kalet, A., Chou, C. (eds.) Boston, MA: Springer, pp. 3–15.

Knobe, M., Munker, R., Sellei, R. M., et al. 2010. Peer teaching: A randomized controlled trial using student-teachers to teach musculoskeletal ultrasound. *Med Educ*, 44, 148–155.

Kogan, L. R., Schoenfeld-Tacher, R., Hellyer, P., et al. 2020. Veterinarians and impostor syndrome: An exploratory study. *Vet Rec*, 187. doi: https://doi.org/10.1136/vr.105914.

Korwin A., Jones, R. 1990. Do hands-on, technology-based activities enhance learning by reinforcing cognitive knowledge and retention? *J Technol Educ*, 1, 26–33.

May, S. 2017. An audience with Stephen May. *Vet Rec*, 181, 162–163.

Malone, E. 2019. Evidence-based clinical skills teaching and learning: What do we really know? *J Vet Med Educ*, 46, 379–398.

Mastenbroek, N. J. J. M., van Beukelen, P., Demerouti, E., et al. 2015. Effects of a 1 year development programme for recently graduated veterinary professionals on personal and job resources: A combined quantitative and qualitative approach. *BMC Vet Res*, 11. doi: https://doi.org/10.1186/s12917-015-0627-y.

Matthew, S. M., Bok, H. G. J., Chaney, K. P., et al. 2020. Collaborative development of a shared framework for competency-based veterinary education. *J Vet Med Educ*, 47, 578–593.

Michels, M. E., Evans, D. E., Bok, G. A. 2012. What is a clinical skill? Searching for order in chaos through a modified Delphi process. *Med Teach*, 34, e573–e581.

Mitchell, S. A., Boyer, T. J. 2020. *Deliberate Practice in Medical Simulation*. Stat Pearls [Internet]. Treasure Island (Fl): Stat Pearls Publishing. January 2020. PMID: 32119445.

Molgaard, L., Read, E. 2017. Peer assisted learning. In: *Veterinary Medical Education: A Practical Guide*. Hodgson, J. L., Pelzer, J. M.

(eds.) Hoboken, NJ: John Wiley & Sons, Inc., pp. 116–129.

Molgaard, L. K., Hodgson, J. L., Bok H. G. J., et al. 2018. *Competency-Based Veterinary Education: Part 1 – CBVE Framework*. Washington, DC: Association of American Veterinary Medical Colleges.

Molgaard, L. K., Chaney, K. P., Bok, H. G. J., et al. 2019. Development of core entrustable professional activities linked to a competency-based veterinary education framework. *Med Teach*, 41, 1404–1410.

Moulton, C. E., Dubrowski, A., MacRae, H., et al. 2006. Teaching surgical skills: What kind of practice makes perfect? A randomized, controlled trial. *Ann Surg*, 244, 400–409.

Moulton, C. E., Regehr, G., Mylopoulos, M., et al. 2007. Slowing down when you should: A new model of expert judgement. *Acad Med*, 82, S109–S116.

Murre, J. M. J. 2014. S-shaped learning curves. *Psychon Bull Rev*, 21, 344–356.

Norcini J., Anderson M. B., Bollela V., et al. 2018. 2018 consensus framework for good assessment. *Med Teach*, 40, 1085–1087.

Oermann, M. H. 2011. Toward evidence-based nursing education: Deliberate practice and motor skill learning. *J Nurs Educ*, 50, 63–64.

Pusic, M., Pecaric, M., Boutis, K. 2011. How much practice is enough? Using learning curves to assess the deliberate practice of radiograph interpretation. *Acad Med*, 86, 31–36.

Pusic, M. V., Boutis, K., Hatala, R., et al. 2015. Learning curves in health professions education. *Acad Med*, 90, 1034–1042.

Pusic, M. V., Boutis, K., Pecaric, M. R., et al. 2017. A primer on the statistical modelling of learning curves in health professions education. *Med Teach*, 22, 741–759.

Pusic, M., Boutis, K., McGaghie, W. C. 2018. Role of scientific theory in simulation education research. *Simul Healthc*, 13, S7–S14.

Read, E. K., Hecker, K. G. 2013. The development and delivery of a systematic veterinary clinical skills education program at the University of Calgary. *J Vet Sci Technol*, S4.

Read, E. K., Brown, A., Maxey, C., et al. 2020. Comparing entrustment and competence: An exploratory look at performance-relevant information in the final year of a veterinary program. *J Vet Med Educ*, Advance On-line. doi: https://doi.org/10.3138/jvme-2019-0128.

Reznick, R. K., MacRae, H. 2006. Teaching surgical skills – changes in the wind. *N Engl J Med*, 355, 2664–2669.

Rothlin, P., Horvath, S., Birrer, D., et al. 2016. Mindfulness promotes the ability to deliver performance in highly demanding situations. *Mindfulness*, 7, 727–733.

Salisbury, S. K., Chaney, K. P., Ilkiw, J. E., et al. 2019. *Competency-Based Veterinary Education: Part 3 - Milestones*. Washington, DC: Association of American Veterinary Medical Colleges.

Salisbury, S. K., Rush, B. R., Ilkiw, J. E., et al. 2020. Collaborative development of core entrustable professional activities for veterinary education. *J Vet Med Educ*, 47, 607–618.

Shea J. B., Morgan R. L. 1979. Contextual interference effects on the acquisition, retention, and transfer of a motor skill. *J Exp Psychol Hum Learn Mem*, 5, 179–187.

Stevens, B., Royal, K. D., Ferris, K., et al. 2019. Effect of a mindfulness exercise on stress in veterinary students performing surgery. *Vet Surg*, 48, 360–366.

Stone, D., Heen, S. 2014. *Thanks for the Feedback: The Science and Art of Receiving Feedback Well (Even When It Is Off base, Unfair, Poorly Delivered, and Frankly, You're Not in the Mood)*. Viking: New York, NY.

Valsamis, E. M., Chouari, T., O'Dowd-Booth, C., et al. 2018. Learning curves in surgery: Variables, analysis and applications. *Postgrad Med J*, 94, 525–530.

Walker M., Peyton J. W. R. 1998. Teaching in the theatre. In: *Teaching and Learning in Medical Practice*. Peyton J. W. R. (ed.) Manticore Europe: Rickmansworth, UK.

Ward, D. S., Zollo, R. 2017. Knowing when to slow down. *Anaesthesia*, 72, 910–924.

Yamada, C., Itaguchi, Y., Fukuzawa, K. 2019. Effects of the amount of practice and time interval between practice sessions on the retention of internal models. *Plos One*, 14, e0215331.

5

How Do I Know if I am Learning What I Need to?

Sheena Warman[1] and Emma K. Read[2]

[1] *Bristol Veterinary School, University of Bristol, Bristol, UK*
[2] *College of Veterinary Medicine, The Ohio State University, Columbus, OH, USA*

Key Messages

- Students are motivated to develop their skills through both summative and formative assessment opportunities, as well as their career aspirations
- Miller's pyramid of clinical competence (knows, knows how, shows, does) creates a useful framework for developing an assessment strategy for clinical skills, carefully aligned with the wider curriculum and opportunities for students to develop their skills further (e.g. in workplace settings)
- Summative assessment tools include Objective Structured Clinical Examination (OSCE) and workplace-based assessments (WBAs), including in-training evaluation reports (ITERs), direct observation of procedural skills (DOPS), mini-clinical evaluation exercise (mini-CEX), case-based discussion (CbD), entrustable professional activities (EPAs), and portfolios

- Effective feedback dialogue is essential to optimize learning, drawing on a range of sources of feedback, and closely integrated with self-assessment and reflection
- A range of frameworks, such as the reflective conversation model, or the "three Ps" approach (in simulation settings) is available to support tutors and learners to develop skills in feedback
- Attention to learner motivation and mindset, supportive tutor–learner relationships, and institutional culture are all critical to ensure that learners fulfil their potential

---

Introduction

Veterinary students are motivated to learn clinical skills for two principle reasons: in the longer term, to ensure they have the skills they will need as practicing professionals and, in the more immediate term, to ensure they pass their skills assessments. In this chapter, we will provide an overview of assessment methods for clinical skills, both in classroom and workplace-based

Veterinary Clinical Skills, First Edition. Edited by Emma K. Read, Matt R. Read, and Sarah Baillie.
© 2022 John Wiley & Sons, Inc. Published 2022 by John Wiley & Sons, Inc.
Companion website: www.wiley.com/go/read/veterinary

settings, and provide some background as to how institutions make decisions about what skills to test, when to test them, and how to test them. We will then consider how students can optimize their learning through the use of feedback, reflection, and coaching.

Why Is Assessing Clinical Skills Important?

In this chapter, we assume a broad definition of "assessment," viewing assessment as any activity that helps a student compare their learning to an expected standard. "Assessment drives learning" is a well-established maxim in education (Watling and Ginsburg, 2019). Traditionally, assessments are considered to primarily have either a *summative* or a *formative* purpose – assessment-*of*-learning or assessment-*for*-learning, respectively (Schuwirth and van der Vleuten, 2011).

"Summative assessment" normally means that the assessment is high stakes, the results of which may contribute to a decision as to whether a student should repeat a unit of teaching or progress further in the program. "Formative assessment" describes assessments designed to support student learning, implying that there will be an opportunity to engage with feedback on a formal or an informal basis during learning or while being assessed performing a clinical skill or procedure. Both summative and formative assessments have a role to play in student development. Summative assessment is important for accreditation of programs and to ensure that professionals graduate with the required skills to enter the workforce, while formative assessment may be used as either a formal part of the curriculum or informally during teaching and work placements, supporting the student as they hone their skills and, ultimately, increasing their chances of success during summative assessments and later in professional life. The boundary between the two types of assessment is often blurred for learners and faculty. Many summative assessments provide opportunities for feedback, and there is a move to programmatic assessment in an increasing number of veterinary and medical schools

where very frequent, low-stakes formative assessments contribute collectively to broader pass–fail decisions (van der Vleuten et al., 2015; van der Vleuten et al., 2018). Programmatic approaches are considered to support a shift from a culture of "grade-chasing" and summative assessment (where feedback can often be overlooked by learners as they focus on "passing") to a culture of individualized learning with a focus on rich narrative feedback, practice, role modeling, and guidance from more experienced tutors. Whether or not there is an explicit strategy of programmatic assessment within a veterinary school, there are often myriad opportunities available for formative assessment and feedback, whether from tutors, clinical staff in the university and on external workplace placement, peers, clients, and even patients themselves, as explored later in this chapter.

Reasons for assessing learning in clinical skills are summarized in Box 5.1. While students will often be motivated to learn clinical skills in order to develop into a competent veterinary professional, it would be naïve of institutions to assume that this alone is enough to drive learning. It is well recognized that assessment is an important

---

Box 5.1 Reasons for Assessing Clinical Skills

Clinical skills can be assessed, formatively and/or summatively, for the following reasons:

- To help students monitor their progress and identify areas of strength and areas for improvement.
- To motivate students to learn and help focus and direct their learning.
- To help tutors identify gaps in teaching, misunderstandings, or areas for improvement.
- To ensure students are meeting standards required by institutions and accrediting bodies.
- To inform and support curriculum and staff development.
- To ensure students are prepared for work placements and clinical rotations.

(if not the most important) driver of individual learning, as well as shaping the broader curriculum (Rust, 2002). For veterinary professionals, it is also important for institutions to be able to demonstrate to accrediting bodies, and the broader public, that their graduating students have achieved the required level of competence. For example, in the United Kingdom, the Royal College of Veterinary Surgeons publishes the "Day One Competences" (RCVS, 2020) and internationally, the American Association of Veterinary Medical Colleges publishes the competency-based veterinary education (CBVE) framework (Molgaard et al., 2019; Matthew, et al., 2020). These wide-ranging frameworks incorporate many clinical skills, such as those relating to patient handling and restraint, clinical examination, sample collection, administration of medication, and basic aseptic surgical skills. The CBVE framework also describes defined clinical activities that a learner must perform during their training program, referred to as entrustable professional activities (EPAs).

Veterinary institutions are accredited by various bodies internationally, for example the American Veterinary Medical Association's Council on Education (AVMA's COE), Royal College of Veterinary Surgeons (RCVS), Australian Veterinary Boards Council (AVBC), and European Association of Establishments for Veterinary Education (EAEVE). Assessment of veterinary programs assures the general public that certain standards are being met during the training of graduates and that students will have a rigorous program that emphasizes the necessary knowledge, skills, values, and attitudes required to be successful in the workplace. Careful construction of assessment and monitoring of learner performance are important aspects of a veterinary program that are scrutinized by accreditors. Assessment of learners informs more than just an individual learner and results of cohorts can be used to provide feedback to teachers and accreditors about the quality of the learning experiences being provided. Accreditation is intended to provide the general public with assurance that

learners are learning what they need to in order to be able to safely and competently perform their job.

Besides assessment, what else motivates students to learn clinical skills? Clinical skills can be taught, learned, rehearsed, and assessed in both classroom and workplace settings. In a carefully structured curriculum, the teaching and assessing of clinical skills will be aligned with opportunities for further practice of skills in workplace settings (McGaghie et al., 2010), creating multiple opportunities for "deliberate practice" (Norman et al., 2018). This can also help motivate students to engage with learning opportunities and focus on skill development. For example, students about to go on a lambing placement might wish to receive formal assessment relating to skills such as basic sheep handling and common lambing presentations to feel assured of their skill level. The students may also be more motivated to rehearse these specific skills in their own time. Students about to go on clinical placements are likely to be motivated to engage with learning relating to the skills and procedures required. Careful alignment of formal teaching and assessments with activities such as work placements can support students to focus on rehearsing essential skills, increasing their confidence such that they can make the most of opportunities to develop their skills further in the workplace setting, on real animals and patients, under the supervision of suitably qualified professionals.

Individual students are also motivated to learn based on their own career aspirations, which can enhance their interest in receiving feedback regarding their own skill level and areas where improvement is required. For example, a student with a strong interest in surgery is likely to find learning basic surgical skills engaging and motivating and they might be driven to practice these skills in order to achieve a higher level of competence than is actually expected at their particular stage of training. Conversely, it can be harder for students to engage with learning skills related to areas they have no interest in, for example learning a skill associated with a species that they have limited experience with or don't anticipate working with following graduation. While the transferable nature of many skills across species, the broad range of competences required by graduates, and the uncertainties of professional life can all be identified as reasons why these skills are important for all students, for some students an underpinning lack of confidence with, or lack of interest in, a particular species can detract from their learning. In these situations, the different interests of students in a cohort can be a powerful resource for engaging students in their own and peer-to-peer learning. For example, a student with significant equine experience who has aspirations of working with horses following graduation can often help support less experienced students to develop confidence with their equine handling skills. In this situation, it may be important to emphasize to all students that, while there are often many variations on how different skills can be performed, for the purposes of assessment, students should focus on those methods taught by the institution. As noted elsewhere, consistent, rigid adherence to a single method of performing a skill is necessary for a novice learner to progress more quickly (Dreyfus and Dreyfus, 1986).

Summative Assessments

Formal assessment of clinical skills can take place within a wide range of formats (Baillie et al., 2014). Miller's pyramid of clinical competence (Figure 5.1) is often used to guide students and faculty through the different levels by which clinical skills can be assessed as a learner progresses through a program of study (Miller, 1990). For example, a student early in the program might be taught knowledge related to suture materials in a lecture setting, which is subsequently assessed using multiple choice questions ("knows"). Next, the student may learn when these different materials are used and what suture patterns might be appropriate ("knows how"). Finally, they may be required to demonstrate their suturing skills on models ("shows"), before finally undertaking suturing on a live patient ("does"). The assessments

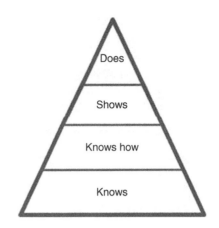

Figure 5.1 Miller's pyramid of clinical competence.

considered in this chapter focus on the "shows" and "does" levels of Miller's pyramid.

A utility formula can be used to help institutions decide on the most appropriate assessments within their settings (van der Vleuten, 1996). This formula considers the reliability, validity, educational impact, acceptability, and cost of different assessments, acknowledging that there is always a degree of compromise when balancing these different qualities. "Reliability" refers broadly to the reproducibility and accuracy of results. "Validity" relates to whether or not the assessment measures what it is supposed to measure. "Educational impact" relates to the influence that the assessment has in shaping students' learning. "Acceptability" refers to whether or not the assessment is perceived as being relevant, engaging, and "acceptable" in the local and wider professional context. Finally, and more than ever, 'cost' is a significant consideration in health professions assessment. Academic, technical, and administrative staff time, room space, technological support, and use of consumables (whether classroom or workplace-based) are significant for any type of clinical skills assessment and need to be factored into any decision relating to what type of assessment will be used.

Within a veterinary training program, there should be a clear strategy for assessing clinical skills, with consideration given to the timing of skills and blueprinting (mapping) those skills back to the overall curriculum. For example, it might be appropriate to schedule assessment of animal handling skills prior to students engaging in farm animal practical experiences or assessment of basic surgical skills before students participate in external rotations in clinical practice. As outlined above, this combination of assessment and upcoming professional learning opportunities can be a powerful motivator for students to engage with learning opportunities and rehearse their skills.

Objective Structured Clinical Examination (OSCE)

OSCEs have been used in medical education for more than four decades (Harden and Gleeson, 1979) and are now widely used in a range of healthcare professions including veterinary medicine. OSCEs assess at the "shows" level of Miller's pyramid of clinical competence. An OSCE consists of multiple mini-stations (ideally between 10 and 20), with different skills or tasks being assessed in each station. Each student rotates through all of the stations in a prescribed sequence, with a standardized amount of time to complete each task, while being assessed using a structured grading system (Dilly and Baillie, 2017). Tasks can vary in complexity depending on the level of training and expected outcomes and can range from basic animal handling skills (e.g. placing a halter on a cow), to performing clinical skills (e.g. suturing, preparing a blood smear, and giving a subcutaneous injection), to demonstrating communication skills (e.g. taking a history from a simulated client). OSCEs take place in a controlled setting and the need for standardization between students often dictates that models are used in place of live animals (Dilly et al., 2016; Dilly and Baillie, 2017). Stations usually last 5–6 minutes for basic tasks such as handwashing or gloving but can take up to 20 minutes for more complex tasks such as history-taking or creation of treatment plans (Baillie et al., 2016).

At each station, the student first reads the provided scenario and background information. The student then enters the station with the examiner and undertakes the task when instructed to do so.

The examiner and student are not normally permitted to talk to one another during the assessment, other than verification of the student's name and confirmation that the student understands the task required. This avoids any tendency for "teaching" during the OSCE, as all students must be treated in the same manner in order to ensure reliability and fairness of assessment. Students are often easily overwhelmed during an OSCE and unclear verbal feedback at one station might affect performance in another station (Baillie et al., 2016).

There are two main approaches to assessment of clinical skill performance with OSCEs: using either a detailed checklist or a global rating scale (GRS). Detailed checklists include a number of anticipated steps ("items") that are part of the procedure (often between 15 and 25), with the examiner determining whether or not the student performed each item and therefore meets the required standard. Most items are equally weighted (i.e. marked as 0 or 1), although there may be some critical steps (e.g. a break in sterility) that carry a heavier weighting or must be completed successfully in order for the station to be passed (i.e. failure to pass that step is an automatic fail for the entire station). The pass mark or minimum performance level (MPL) can be set in advance of the OSCE being completed ("a priori") or after all of the students have taken it ("post hoc").

For small-to-medium class sizes, the MPL can be determined using standard setting techniques such as modified Angoff or Ebel weighting, whereby a panel of experts in the skill being assessed makes educated estimates of student performance on each item before the exam is given. Since these estimates are being used to establish an MPL, it is important that assessors base their "estimates" on the abilities of a "minimally performing student" and not on the abilities of an average student.

The second approach to determining the MPL is to administer the OSCE and then calculate the pass mark using a borderline regression or borderline group method (Boursicot et al., 2007). This is more frequently used with larger cohorts and occurs after the exam is given so that the performance of students is already known. More on these methods and how to use them is discussed in Chapter 6.

Students' clinical skills performance may also be assessed using a GRS type of form, in which the items are grouped together to create broader categories such as safety, time, and motion or manual dexterity. Typically, there are 4–8 categories for each skill, and an examiner assesses a student in each category using an anchored Likert scale. Research suggests that simple checklists (above) are more useful and appropriate for assessing simple skills and novice learners, but as learners become more proficient (i.e. in later years of the program), GRS scoring provides an increased ability to differentiate an individual's performance within the station and provide more specific feedback for performance improvement (Read et al., 2015).

The reliability of OSCEs is enhanced through the careful piloting of the scenarios and their associated marking sheets; close communication between station authors, examiners, and instructors; formal examiner training; and post-examination analysis of inter-examiner reliability. Student briefing is also essential for reducing anxiety and ensuring that they have an understanding of how the examination will operate (Hecker et al., 2010; Hecker et al., 2012a). Consideration should also be given as to whether to release the titles (or topics) of the stations prior to the examination. While students strongly desire to know exactly what skills to practice for the exam, prior knowledge of the stations may mean students will not take the opportunity to practice a broad range of skills and will only study "to the test." If stations are not formally announced but are delivered over multiple days due to a large cohort size, then students on later days are likely to be perceived as having an unfair advantage because they can quickly review those specific skills.

Feedback from OSCE examinations that is provided to learners varies between institutions. It is common to provide cohort-level (whole class) feedback to a group of students, outlining what was generally done well and highlighting common errors that may have been observed. In some cases, this involves class meetings and verbal feedback from examiners, and in other cases, this involves publishing the exam results for the class and comparing them to previous classes. Individualized (student) feedback can be provided by giving students access to the checklists and/or any written comments from examiners. It should be noted that there is usually very limited time available for examiners to record comments during the exam itself, so comments may be limited or somewhat difficult to interpret out of context by learners. As a result, it can therefore be difficult for a student to correlate the feedback that was written down on the scoring sheet with the overall pass/fail decision for that station. Students need to be informed about this difficulty before being given access to raw checklists in order to avoid them arguing about individual points and failing to focus on whether or not they can actually "do" the skill efficiently and effectively.

Workplace-Based Assessments

Veterinary education has started to adopt the wide range of workplace-based assessments (WBAs) that are used in other health professions to our own unique needs (Magnier and Pead, 2017). These types of assessments are used in the clinical or veterinary workplace in real time and involve a combination of formative and summative tools. They assess at the level of "does" in Miller's pyramid of clinical competence, meaning that they focus on actual cases in a real practice setting (Magnier and Pead, 2017). Unlike OSCEs that use contrived settings and scenarios, WBAs allow a learner to receive feedback on their ability to perform as a veterinarian while being supervised under the license of a qualified individual. Assessments of this type include in-training evaluation reports (ITERs), direct observation of procedural skills (DOPS), mini-clinical evaluation exercise (mini-CEX), and case-based discussion (CbD).

EPAs have recently been described as a further opportunity for using some of these assessment tools, while not actually being an assessment themselves. EPAs describe routine everyday activities that can be entrusted to a learner when they are ready and allow for observation so that a learner's skills can be evaluated using some type of WBA.

WBAs lend themselves to a programmatic approach in which individual assessments may be considered relatively "low-stakes" and can be primarily formative in nature, but when all of the individual assessments are aggregated, it can lead to an overall summative pass/fail decision. WBA tools can also be incorporated into students' portfolios, often with the addition of written self-reflection that may subsequently be reviewed by a coaching or competence committee (Rich et al., 2020). Recent models of programmatic assessment include two parts: a "production cycle" where the student is assessed and a "use cycle" where the feedback is reviewed (Rich et al., 2020).

In-training Evaluation Reports (ITERs)

Traditionally, clinical students in veterinary medicine have received written reports of their performance at the end of each rotation or experience. Ideally, students should also receive feedback in the middle of the rotation so as to alert them to problem areas that might need fixing before completion of the learning opportunity. Research in other health professions has shown the importance of training assessors prior to them providing feedback on ITERs, as well as reporting on the "hidden" meaning that often inadvertently occurs with written feedback forms (Dudek et al., 2008; Ginsburg et al., 2017). ITERs are intended to provide feedback to a student regarding development across various competencies in a framework and have traditionally been scored on a Likert scale using subjective anchors. More recently, milestones have been developed to help identify the developmental stages needed as a student progresses toward competence and these may also help provide language for clinicians to guide learning feedback, as well as to determine when learners are ready to move on to the next stage of training (Salisbury et al., 2019). While ITERs remain an important tool for determining a student's overall progress in the clinic, they are not timely and are primarily only used for summative feedback. For these reasons, ITERs are now frequently being supplemented with other WBAs as programmatic assessment becomes more commonplace and demands multiple "snapshots" of learner performance for a more complete picture of the student's abilities to be formed (Norcini et al., 2018).

Direct Observation of Procedural Skills (DOPS)

DOPS are used to evaluate performance of practical skills in a clinical workplace setting (Hecker et al., 2012b; Magnier et al., 2012; Weijs et al., 2015). In this case, a learner is observed performing a clinical skill and is scored by an assessor who has expertise in that practice area. It is normal for a range of skills to be identified and assessed over a specified time period. In veterinary education, attention must be paid to the species and settings within which different skills can be assessed, mapping this to the students' work placements. Examples of standardized forms that can be used to document these assessments are available in the literature (Wilkinson et al., 2008). To increase the reliability of assessing a single skill (and given the range of situations encountered in the workplace, e.g. different animal temperaments and anatomy), individual skills should ideally be observed/assessed multiple times over the course of training (i.e. a minimum of six is suggested). However, this has significant resource implications that may not be achievable across multiple skills within a veterinary hospital setting. An alternative approach is to require the students to request assessment when they consider themselves to have reached the required standard and feel ready to be evaluated. This self-assessment acts as the "gate-keeper" to ensure the likelihood of summative assessment at a time when the student has acquired some competence and confidence in their skill. It is important that both the assessor and the student understand that the student must ask to be evaluated prior to beginning the procedure, because retrospective assessment of a successful procedure is not appropriate and may lead to omissions in detail. One of the major advantages of using DOPS is the opportunity to provide the student with structured, formative, in-the-moment feedback, albeit linked to a summative assessment. Challenges include ensuring that there are sufficient opportunities for all students to rehearse and be assessed on each skill within the required time frame and ensuring adequate staff and student training in the process of using this type of assessment.

Mini-Clinical Evaluation Exercise (mini-CEX)

The mini-CEX involves direct observation of a learner by one assessor during a routine patient/client encounter in a typical clinical setting (Hecker et al., 2012b; Magnier et al., 2012; Weijs et al., 2015). An example of this type of encounter in veterinary practice may be an initial consultation with a client. The observation normally lasts 15–20 minutes and is typically followed by immediate feedback from the assessor (Norcini, 2005). Performance on a list of skills required as part of the task is rated using a range of descriptors such as "below," "at," or "above" expectations. This feedback can then be used to develop an action plan for further improvement. As previously described, to enhance the overall reliability of the assessment, observation and evaluation of multiple encounters (usually 6–8) is required.

Case-based Discussion (CbD)

A CbD is a formal discussion between a learner and their assessor regarding a clinical case, usually lasting around 20 minutes followed by 5 minutes or so of feedback discussion. In medicine, CbDs are normally used at postgraduate level, where the learner has been directly responsible for case management (Setna et al., 2010). Although discussion focuses on a specific case that was encountered during clinical work, the discussion itself usually takes place in a room that allows for some privacy (e.g. an office or meeting room). CbDs are usually used for formative assessment, although they may also contribute to a portfolio or programmatic assessment approach. During the discussion, the learner has access to the case records while the assessor probes their level of understanding, decision-making, and clinical judgment. There should be an opportunity to reflect on the decisions that were made, as well as a discussion of concerns that arose. A structured assessment form is used to capture evaluation of a range of skills such as prioritizing information, planning, and record-keeping. Examples of forms used in postgraduate medical training are available (e.g. https://www.iscp.ac.uk/static/public/cbd_form.pdf). The discussion is followed by verbal "in-the-moment" feedback, usually summarized on the assessment form. In a similar manner to mini-CEX, multiple CbDs should be undertaken over a period of training, reflecting the range of types of cases for which the learner is responsible.

Entrustable Professional Activities (EPAs)

EPAs are routine tasks that are part of daily practice and incorporate multiple competencies simultaneously. To clarify, competencies describe the veterinarian and what they can do, whereas EPAs describe the work that a veterinarian does that requires integration of those competencies (Molgaard et al., 2019).

EPAs can be delegated to a learner who has reached a certain level of training and is expected to be able to perform them independently (or as much as they can practice independently). In veterinary medicine, learners are never licensed to practice on their own prior to graduation, whereas in medicine, EPAs are used with learners that are already licensed to practice independently and are working at a graduate level (ten Cate and Taylor, 2020).

In this scenario, the observing clinician watches the learner perform the EPA and either assesses them using the WBA tools already described above or an "entrustment scale" (also referred to as an *entrustability scale* or an *entrustment-supervision scale*) (ten Cate et al., 2020). There are various types of entrustment scales, and it is not yet clear which are the most efficacious (ten Cate et al., 2020). There is much ongoing debate on this topic, and EPAs are currently a focus of a multi-institution, international study in veterinary medicine being conducted by the American Association of Veterinary Medical Colleges' Council on Outcomes-based Veterinary Education (COVE), formerly known as CBVE (https://urldefense. com/v3/__https://www.aavmc__;!!N11eV2 iwtfs!-OPkIUUzau8sJdZvVgEFLIQhP3CMtyoo Gey1HwMB772MxxRoi3gTE3UsLn2XNewO$. org/news/vet-med-educator-august-2020/). The currently described entrustment scales focus on various different aspects of practice: what a learner is able to do by themself (e.g. "Learner could not perform and had to observe only") (Rekman et al., 2016), what the supervisor had to do (e.g. "I had to prompt them from time to time") (Gofton et al., 2012), and to what degree the supervisor feels they could entrust the learner to perform the task the next time they are asked to do it (e.g. "Trust with on-demand guidance") (ten Cate et al., 2016; Chen and ten Cate, 2018). Entrustment scales may also be differentiated according to whether they are *retrospective* (i.e. how much supervision was actually provided during performance?) versus *prospective* (i.e. how much supervision will be required in the near future?) (ten Cate et al., 2020).

Use of EPAs and entrustment scales as types of assessment form has just started in veterinary medicine. The CBVE framework describes eight EPAs that were developed by consensus across all of the AAVMC veterinary colleges and efforts are underway to explore entrustment scale use for assessment of those EPAs (Molgaard et al., 2019; Salisbury et al., 2020). Pilot use of entrustment was conducted across practices in a distributed final-year education model and showed that comments on entrustment scale scores were more learner specific, longer in length, and used more of a coaching voice than feedback provided on ITER evaluations (Read et al., 2020). Clinicians described entrustment scales as being easy to use, and there was less need for formal training of the assessors. These attributes could be advantageous in a distributed-teaching environment where it can be difficult to provide outreach to all assessors in a timely manner or in a busy, yet understaffed, teaching hospital where training time is often impractical (Read et al., 2020). More work is yet to be done to validate the use of entrustment scales in veterinary education.

Portfolios

Portfolios are increasingly being used in veterinary education to provide an opportunity for students to collate multiple pieces of coursework and WBAs, accompanied by written reflection on their progress. Whether they are paper based or online, portfolios are a tool for integrating assessments in a holistic manner and they support students as they reflect on their longitudinal progress during their training and identify any recurring areas of strength or priorities for improvement. While portfolios often contain multiple individual assessments such as DOPS, mini-CEX, and CbDs, the portfolio itself can be assessed in a summative manner, usually by committee review.

There is much evidence that portfolios have far more learning value if the reflective writing is supported by face-to-face discussion with a trusted supervisor (e.g. a personal tutor) (Driessen, 2017; Warman, 2020). Writing purely for summative purposes, where reflective writing is reviewed by an assessor but there is no opportunity to have a formative discussion with the student, can lead students to play "the reflective game" whereby they simply write what they think an assessor might want to read in order to judge their competence, rather than reflecting in a constructive manner that would be more likely to lead to meaningful insights and action planning for further development (Warman, 2020).

Making the Most of Feedback

What Is Feedback and How Useful Is It?

Feedback in clinical education has been defined as "specific information about the comparison between a trainee's observed performance and a standard, given with the intent to improve the trainee's performance" (van de Ridder et al., 2008). Feedback during clinical training is likely to encompass a combination of "in-the-moment" feedback during or following a procedure (whether in the classroom or clinic), scheduled feedback or debriefing sessions during or following a placement, and written feedback relating to coursework, assessments, or placements (Warman et al., 2014a).

Traditional views of feedback conceptualize it as a one-way flow of information from a teacher to a learner. However, more recently, our understanding of feedback centers on the role of the learner in seeking and using feedback, highlighting the importance of dialogue and trust between tutor and learner (Archer, 2010; Murdoch-Eaton, 2012; Molloy and Boud, 2013; Ramani et al., 2019a). Many studies have explored the effect of feedback on learning, with meta-analyses showing a variable but generally moderate beneficial effect (Kluger and DeNisi, 1996; Issenberg et al., 2005; Hatala et al., 2014; van de Ridder et al., 2015). These studies indicate that feedback has the potential to be a powerful influencer of learning, but it must be used carefully and strategically to optimize this potential and reduce the risk of it having a deleterious effect on learning. For example, feedback can be more effective for improving the performance of the learner when the learner initially has a low skill level, there is purposeful setting of goals, and the feedback message itself is encouraging, specific, and frequent (van de Ridder et al., 2015). Without feedback, mistakes are likely to go uncorrected, good practice unrecognized, and clinical competence achieved by good fortune or not at all (Ende, 1983).

If learning a new skill relies solely on self-assessment (which is often inaccurate), a lack of insight into errors leads learners to overestimate their competence (Kruger and Dunning, 1999; Davis et al., 2006; Ramani et al., 2017a). Reflection and feedback, two closely related concepts, are essential for enabling further development of skills (Sargeant et al., 2009). The literature suggests a wide range of factors that can be harnessed to increase the effectiveness of feedback. While many studies focus on the process of feedback, more recently the role of the learner, their relationship with the feedback giver, and the wider institutional culture have been highlighted. Each of these is considered later in this chapter.

Potential Sources of Feedback

There are many potential sources of feedback when learning clinical skills, and there is evidence that harnessing a wide range of sources leads to more effective learning (Hatala et al., 2014, Fenwick and Dahlgren, 2015). Feedback can come not just from tutors but also from peers, simulators, and patients and can be integrated with the learner's own reflection and self-assessment. Peers, often with a range of prior experiences, can provide one another with feedback on basic skills, often in the context of a trusted peer relationship. Simulated clients, often used in the teaching of communication skills, can provide invaluable feedback from the perspective of animal owners (Mossop et al., 2015). Veterinary patients themselves, through their reactions and behavior, can let a learner know whether their technique is effective and minimize discomfort. Models and simulators can be designed to provide feedback to the user. For example, a haptic model used to teach bovine rectal palpation skills was designed to give an audible "moo" if a learner exerts excessive pressure, and a hand hygiene training model provides learners with immediate feedback on their technique (Baillie et al., 2008; Mosley et al., 2019).

Being open and alert to different kinds of feedback from a wide range of sources is invaluable in supporting learning. Frequent, concurrent feedback for learning of skills such as ovariohysterectomy can be facilitated by an adequate tutor–learner ratio, made easier by using a classroom setup that facilitates a closer relationship between individual tutors and learners, helping the tutor to identify students who may need more support (Williamson et al., 2019).

Frameworks for Feedback

For feedback to be effective, it should be timely, constructive, specific, actionable, and aligned with the learner's needs (Watling, 2014; Lefroy et al., 2015). Wherever possible, it should be based on direct observation by the tutor (i.e. so it is "owned" by the person offering the feedback). Key features of effective feedback, tailored to the clinical workplace, are summarized in Box 5.2 (Ramani and Krackov, 2012; Warman et al., 2014a).

When learning clinical skills, feedback can be concurrent with, or happen after, the learning event. There is evidence that feedback at the end of the event is more effective for relatively simple tasks, with feedback being offered during the event itself being more beneficial for the learning of more complex tasks (Hatala et al., 2014).

Box 5.2   Key Considerations for Effective Feedback in Clinical Settings

- Knowledge of expected standards: both the learner and tutor should be aware of the expected standards, appropriate to the stage of training
- Feedback should happen at an appropriate time and place: feedback conversations should normally happen as soon as possible after the learning event. Most conversations can be held in front of peers, in a supportive and constructive manner, unless the tutor anticipates that the learner will find the conversation particularly challenging
- Learners should be encouraged to reflect on and evaluate their own performance. Frameworks such as the reflective conversation model can support this
- Feedback should be accurate and owned: students usually reject feedback that they consider inaccurate or unreliable. Wherever possible, the feedback conversation should be with a tutor who directly observed the performance
- Feedback should be objective and non-judgmental. It should give constructive advice on improving specific behaviors and not directly criticize the learner's personal qualities and attributes
- Feedback should be specific. It is much more valuable to give specific examples of what went well or needs to be improved, rather than generic statements such as "well done" or "keep practicing"
- Feedback should be balanced and supportive. Both strengths and weaknesses (framed as areas for improvement or growth) should be discussed. Attention should be paid to body language and any perception of hierarchy between the tutor and learner. A student will value feedback more when he/she perceives that the tutor has the student's best interests at heart
- Ensure an achievable action plan. Without an action plan, feedback can become meaningless. Supporting the student to propose an achievable action plan, focusing on one or two specific goals, is invaluable
- Create ongoing opportunities. Students should be supported to identify and use opportunities for practicing specific skills. It may be that specific aspects of skills (e.g. syringe handling as part of blood sampling) can be rehearsed prior to the next opportunity with models or patients
- Develop a feedback culture. Feedback is a skill that both learners and tutors can rehearse and hone. A collaborative learning culture normalizes supportive feedback conversations

Source: Warman et al., 2014a.

For more complex simulations, such as a team approach to a cardiopulmonary resuscitation scenario, the importance of providing feedback from a range of sources in the context of a team debrief is constructive (McGaghie et al., 2010).

A wide range of models to structure feedback conversations are available, such as "Pendleton's rules" (Pendleton et al., 1984), the agenda-led outcomes-based analysis (ALOBA) model (Silverman et al., 1996; Chowdhury and Kalu, 2004), and a coaching-based framework "R2C2" discussed in more detail later in this chapter (Sargeant et al., 2015, Sargeant et al., 2018). The authors' preference is to use a reflective conversation model, building on Pendleton's rules. This model can also be adapted to draw on aspects of the ALOBA model and is described further below.

A focus on reflection is central to ensuring that feedback will be effective (Sargeant et al., 2009). Reflection is traditionally viewed as an internal, individual process. However, this method has significant limitations: accurate self-assessment of skills is challenging for novices (Kruger and Dunning, 1999), emotional reactions to feedback can limit the acceptance of feedback from others (Sargeant et al., 2008; Bok et al., 2013), and it can be difficult to convert a tendency to worry into purposeful outcomes (Warman, 2020). Understanding reflection as an inherently social process can support more purposeful, productive reflection (Boud et al., 2006). Facilitating reflection through feedback dialogue, with a focus on strengths, weaknesses, and action plans can support the learner to acknowledge and integrate the perspectives of others into their own self-assessment, supporting lifelong learning and development.

While the 'reflective conversation' model is a pragmatic approach to feedback dialogue between a learner and a tutor, it can also be used to facilitate peer-to-peer feedback. The conversation is framed by three questions: (i) *what went well*, (ii) *what went less well* (or what could be improved), and (iii) *what action plan can be identified for improvement*. During each phase, the tutor uses these questions (para-phrased to suit their own style) to invite the learner to reflect on their own performance, with discussion supported and enriched by the observations of the tutor. The learner should generally contribute at least half of the discussion during the conversation.

Advantages of this model are that it is straightforward and easy to implement; it encourages reflection on both strengths and weaknesses, prioritizes an action plan and any concerns of the learner, is applicable to a wide range of settings, and can be very time-efficient. Challenges include a tendency of learners to want to jump straight to consideration of what could have been done differently or better, rather than start with a focus on strengths. Sometimes, the framework can be perceived as formulaic or even patronizing, but the risk of this is minimized with care to phrasing of questions and developing a trusting relationship between learner and tutor.

The framework can often be enhanced by using aspects of the agenda-led model – before the task is undertaken, the learner is asked to identify any areas they would particularly value feedback on and what they want to focus on as an outcome during the task. The reflective conversation can then focus on discussion of specific aspects of performance that can be further developed in order to achieve the desired outcome.

In simulation settings, a "three Ps" approach has also been described: planning, pre-briefing, and providing the feedback (Motola et al., 2013). The planning step involves consideration of how and when feedback should be integrated within the session. Pre-briefing allows any rules and expectations to be explained and highlights the importance of a nonthreatening, confidential, and safe environment. Feedback can then be provided both during the simulation and as a post-event debrief. A plus/delta (+/Δ) framework for debriefing can be used, with similarities to the reflective conversation model described above (Motola et al., 2013). Two columns (+ and Δ) are created on a whiteboard or flipchart paper, with participants brainstorming what went well (+) and what could be changed (i.e.

weaknesses and suggestions for improvement (Δ). This framework allows for structured, reflective, time-efficient debriefing, giving the facilitator an opportunity to focus on a few key learning points identified from the participant's reactions and reflection.

The Role of the Learner

While most students understand that feedback is an integral part of learning, engaging with feedback can be an emotional process (Sargeant et al., 2008; Eva et al., 2012; Bok et al., 2013). Well-intentioned, specific, accurate feedback is useless if it is not well-received and engaged with to inform an action plan. Some of the ways in which learners can optimize their use of feedback are identified below (van der Leeuw and Slootweg, 2013).

- Take your time: time can help separate emotions from the content of feedback, enabling you to see the value of the feedback more clearly.
- Read feedback carefully, looking for common themes across different pieces of feedback.
- Find a balance between being self-confident and humble when engaging with feedback.
- Keep your professional goals in mind, and consider the perspectives of your teachers as they support you to reach these.
- Talk about feedback with your teachers and peers.
- Foster a love of learning – use your feedback to create personal learning plans to put feedback into action.

This last point can be considered from the perspective of mindset, as was mentioned in Chapter 4. Dweck describes two types of mindset: a *fixed mindset* (performance goal orientation) and a *growth mindset* (learning goal orientation) (Dweck, 2000; Dweck, 2012). Learners with a fixed mindset believe that intelligence and ability are innate and can't be developed, they feel threatened by failure, and they may be more likely to reject constructive feedback (Teunissen et al., 2009). Learners with a growth mindset believe that hard work and practice are central to success and that failure is part of learning. Mindset is of itself not considered to be innate – it is formed from early childhood through our interactions with others, it evolves over time, and it can be shaped and changed throughout our lives, both through our own efforts and the influence of those with whom we interact. In veterinary medicine, a growth mindset has been linked with improved well-being (Root Kustritz, 2017; Whittington et al., 2017) and with reduced anxiety regarding clinical rotation teaching, with clinicians being viewed as future colleagues rather than intimidating teachers (Bostock et al., 2018).

Fostering a Collaborative Learning Culture

In the last decade or so, research relating to assessment and feedback has shifted in its perspective from having a focus on an individual's learning to the wider learning culture. This shift draws on sociocultural theories of learning, where an individual's learning is not solely the product of their own mind and endeavors but is fostered and shaped as learners become integrated within their professional community. Understanding how a community's values and practices influence individual learning yields valuable insights into ways of supporting learners and fostering culture of collaborative learning (Watling and Ginsburg, 2019). There is much that can be learnt from the world of music and sports, where the perceived credibility of a teacher or coach is influenced not just by their technical skills but by their instructional abilities (Watling et al., 2014).

Fostering supportive relationships and creating a safe learning environment are essential skills for tutors. Feedback can be an emotional process. Constructive feedback should focus on the task itself (i.e. task-oriented) rather than making judgments about the learner (i.e. person-oriented). Uptake and engagement with feedback are reduced if the feedback threatens the learner's self-esteem or triggers strong negative emotions (Sargeant et al., 2008; Eva et al., 2012; Bok et al., 2013). Learners make choices about what feedback they engage with and find to be credible. Learners may sense conflicting feedback and cues from tutors, peers, clients, and patients, and they may choose to reject feedback that is overly challenging to their sense of self or is from a source that is perceived as being less credible. There are several factors that are key to establishing a collaborative feedback culture (Warman et al., 2014b; Ramani et al., 2017b; Ramani et al., 2019a) including the encouragement of feedback seeking and engagement with feedback, supported by positive relationships between the learner and tutor set within a wider culture of collaborative learning.

Feedback-seeking behavior has been studied in the veterinary clinical setting (Bok et al., 2013), uncovering a range of personal and interpersonal influences on a student's willingness to seek feedback. As outlined above, a student's mindset and personal goals play roles in engagement with feedback, as do the perceived credibility of the tutor, and the relationship between learner and tutor. Additionally, students might weigh up the anticipated pros and cons to seeking feedback in relation to the potential emotional cost (e.g. risk of negative feelings if feedback is critical) or risks to their image in front of their peers, clients, and supervisors. They may prioritize protecting their sense of self or image over risking critical comments from a supervisor. This concept of "feedback profit" requires attention to the wider culture of learning and feedback. It is also recognized that some learning opportunities may trigger anxious feelings in students, so a supportive climate and constructive feedback is essential to ensuring that students gain optimal learning from these opportunities (Langebaek et al., 2012).

However, a culture of "niceness" can also be detrimental to feedback (Ramani et al., 2017b; Watling and Ginsburg, 2019). A fear of upsetting students can lead faculty to provide written or verbal feedback that is bland and generic, lacking the specificity and guidance required to support development. Overcoming this tension requires attention to staff and student training, trusting relationships, and a climate of collaborative learning.

To foster the optimal feedback climate, tutors and supervisors must work to provide a positive learning culture that fosters a growth mindset. Ramani (2019b) describes steps that learners, teachers, and institutions can take:

- Learners can develop an awareness of their own mindset tendencies and consciously try to adopt a more growth-focused approach, seeking and engaging with feedback and using it to develop action plans.
- Teachers can role-model feedback seeking, welcoming multiple perspectives and acknowledging their own limitations and weaknesses, and focusing feedback conversations on observed behaviors and goals. These actions can help foster a positive learning climate with a culture of mutual respect. Through feedback conversations that focus on observed behaviors and goals, facilitating student reflection, and supported self-assessment, growth mindsets can be nurtured in students.
- Working together, learners and teachers can establish an educational alliance through constructive feedback dialogue, rather than one-way flows of information. Learners and teachers can work together to create opportunities for further learning and putting action plans into place.
- Institutions can support a focus on constructive feedback as part of a climate of assessment for learning to promote professional development at all levels, establish a culture of continuous improvement, support a balance between learner supervision and autonomy, and emphasize a culture of feedback and coaching that enhances professional growth.

One model that institutions, teachers, and learners can use to help foster a culture of feedback is the "Johari Window," a psychological matrix that enables an understanding of our own behaviors, feelings, and motivations during interactions with others (Luft, 1969; Ramani et al., 2017a), helping foster a collaborative culture of self-assessment, reflection, and feedback.

The Johari window has four quadrants, each representing a different level of self-awareness (see Figure 5.2). The "known" quadrant is the most productive in terms of development, fostering a growth mindset through facilitated discussion of strengths and weaknesses. The "blind" quadrant requires careful negotiation. Constructive, reflective feedback conversations can help a learner acknowledge their blind spots. However, learners with a fixed mindset or performance goal approach may find this particularly challenging to their sense of self and may resist seeking feedback and fail to acknowledge its credibility or significance. The "hidden" quadrant relates to concerns or fears that a learner is unwilling to disclose to their tutor. Uncovering this quadrant usually requires the establishment and development of a trusting relationship, which can be challenging in the context of low staff:student ratios and short clinical placements. Role modeling by staff and making their own uncertainty and fears explicit can help to foster a culture that encourages admission of limitations. The "unknown" quadrant can be the most challenging. Alternative perspectives can often provide useful insight so seeking opinions of clients and other professionals can be helpful.

The Role of Coaching

There are challenges for tutors and learners around the tension between assessment *of* learning and assessment *for* learning. Many times, particularly in clinical environments, the same tutors are involved in both training and assessment, often concurrently. In classroom settings, the same staff are often responsible for both fostering a supportive learning climate during timetabled teaching and assessing students during practical examinations. Notwithstanding this tension, arising from the impact of a need for robust assessment of competence and the nuances that it brings to a tutor–learner relationship, there is increasing evidence that fostering a culture of coaching is beneficial to the development of clinical skills. Coaches build longitudinal relationships with students, supporting them to engage with, integrate, and plan from assessment information and multiple sources of feedback. This may be particularly relevant to the veterinary clinical skills context, where clinical skills teachers are recognized as crucial to student learning, teaching students across multiple years and in a wide range of skills and revision sessions (Dilly et al., 2016; Dilly and Baillie, 2017).

The terminology of coaching itself has value; a narrative of "coaching" feels very different to staff and students compared to one of "assessment" (Watling and Ginsburg, 2019). For coaching to have significant impact, time and training need to be committed. With the development of trusting longitudinal relationships, learners may be more inclined to process and engage with challenging feedback, and more likely to develop and follow through on appropriate action plans, supporting the development of a growth mindset to support their lifelong learning.

The R2C2 model draws on sociocultural theories and provides an alternative structure for facilitated reflective feedback conversations and has been shown to improve acceptance and uptake of feedback (Sargeant et al., 2015; Sargeant et al., 2018). The model has four phases: (i) building *rapport* and *relationship*; (ii) exploring *reaction* to, and perceptions of, the data/report; (iii) exploring student (physician) understanding of the *content* of the data/report; and (iv) *coaching* for performance change. Each phase is moderated through facilitated reflection

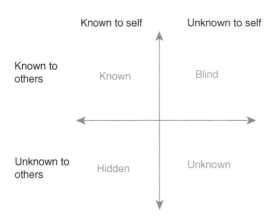

Figure 5.2 The Johari Window (see text for explanation).

on the feedback data and discussion of what it means to the learner. The guiding aim of the model is to empower the learner to embrace ownership of their feedback and performance data and take responsibility for its use to inform their future development.

Conclusion

Effective assessment of clinical skills, closely integrated with the wider curriculum, is essential to ensure that learners develop the clinical and practical skills they will need in their professional lives. Both institutions and students have a responsibility to ensure that essential skills are taught, rehearsed, and assessed. Institutions have a responsibility to their students, accreditors, and the wider public, and students have responsibility to themselves, their future employers and patients, and the wider profession. A supportive culture of effective feedback dialogue, aligned with a robust assessment strategy, can help achieve these goals.

References

Archer, J. C. 2010. State of the science in health professional education: Effective feedback. *Med Educ*, 44, 101–108.

Baillie, S., Crossan, A., Forrest, N., et al. 2008. Developing the "Ouch-o-Meter" to teach safe and effective use of pressure for palpation. In: *Haptics: Perception, Devices and Scenarios. EuroHaptics 2008. Lecture Notes in Computer Science*, Vol. 5024. Ferre, M. (ed.) Berlin Heidelberg: Springer.

Baillie, S., Warman, S. M., Rhind, S. M. 2014. *A Guide to Assessment in Veterinary Medical Education*, 2nd Edition. Bristol: University of Bristol.

Baillie, S., Booth, N., Catterall, A. et al. 2016. A Guide to Veterinary Clinical Skills Laboratories. http://www.bris.ac.uk/vetscience/media/docs/csl-guide.pdf Accessed October 1, 2021.

Bok, H. G. J., Teunissen, P. W., Spruijt, A., et al. 2013. Clarifying students' feedback-seeking behaviour in clinical clerkships. *Med Educ*, 47, 282–291.

Bostock, R., Kinnison, T. May, S. A. 2018. Mindset and its relationship to anxiety in clinical veterinary students. *Vet Rec*, 183, 623.

Boud, D., Cressey, P., Docherty, P. (eds.) 2006. *Productive Reflection at Work*. Abingdon, Oxon: Routledge.

Boursicot, K., Roberts, T., Pell, G. 2007. Using borderline methods to compare passing standards for OSCEs at graduation across three medical schools. *Med Educ*, 41, 1024–1031.

Chen, H. C., ten Cate, O. 2018. Assessment through entrustable professional activities. In: *Learning and Teaching in Clinical Contexts: A Practial Guide*. Delany, C., Molloy, E. (eds.) Chatswood, Australia: Elsevier.

Chowdhury, R. R., Kalu, G. 2004. Learning to give feedback in medical education. *Obstet Gynaecol*, 6, 243–247.

Davis, D. A., Mazmanian, P. E., Fordis, M., et al. 2006. Accuracy of physician self-assessment compared with observed measures of competence: A systematic review. *J Am Med Assoc*, 296, 1094–1102.

Dilly, M., Read, E. K. Baillie, S. 2016. A survey of established veterinary clinical skills laboratories from Europe and North America: Present practices and recent developments. *J Vet Med Educ*, 44, 580–589.

Dilly, M., Baillie, S. 2017. Learning and teaching in clinical skills laboratories. In: *Veterinary Medical Education: A Practical Guide*. Hodgson, J., Pelzer, J. (eds.) Hoboken, NJ: Wiley and Sons, Inc.

Dreyfus, H. L., Dreyfus, S. E. 1986. *Mind Over Machine: The Power of Human Intuition and Expertise in the Era of the Computer*. New York: Free Press.

Driessen, E. 2017. Do portfolios have a future? *Adv Health Sci Educ Theory Pract*, 22, 221–228.

Dudek, N. L., Marks, M. B., Woods, T. J., et al. 2008. Assessing the quality of supervisors' completed clinical evaluation reports. *Med Educ*, 42, 816–822.

Dweck, C. S. 2000. *Self-Theories: Their Role in Motivation, Personality and Development.* Philadelphia: Psychology Press.

Dweck, C. S. 2012. *Mindset: How You Can Fulfil Your Potential.* New York: Ballantine.

Ende, J. 1983. Feedback in clinical medical education. *J Am Med Assoc*, 250, 777–781.

Eva, K. W., Armson, H., Holmboe, E., et al. 2012. Factors influencing responsiveness to feedback: On the interplay between fear, confidence, and reasoning processes. *Adv Health Sci Educ Theory Pract*, 17, 15–26.

Fenwick, T., Dahlgren, M. A. 2015. Towards socio-material approaches in simulation-based education: lessons from complexity theory. *Med Educ*, 49, 359–367.

Ginsburg, S., van der Vleuten, C., Eva, K., et al. 2017. Cracking the code: resident interpretations of written assessment comments. *Med Educ*, 51, 401–410.

Gofton, W. T., Dudek, N. L., Wood, T. J., et al. 2012. The Ottawa Surgical Competency Operating Room Evaluation (O-SCORE): A tool to assess surgical competence. *Acad Med*, 87, 1401–1407.

Harden, R. M., Gleeson, F. A. 1979. Assessment of clinical competence using an objective stuctured clinical examination (OSCE). *Med Educ*, 13, 41–54.

Hatala, R., Cook, D. A., Zendejas, B., et al. 2014. Feedback for simulation-based procedural skills training: A meta-analysis and critical narrative synthesis. *Adv Health Sci Educ Theory Pract*, 19, 251–272.

Hecker, K., Read, E. K., Vallevand, A., et al. 2010. Assessment of first-year veterinary students' clinical skills using objective structured clinical examinations. *J Vet Med Educ*, 37, 395–402.

Hecker, K. G., Adams, C. L., Coe, J. B. 2012a. Assessment of first-year veterinary students' communication skills using an objective structured clinical examination: The importance of context. *J Vet Med Educ*, 39, 304–310.

Hecker, K. G., Norris, J., Coe, J. B. 2012b. Workplace-based assessment in a primary-care setting. *J Vet Med Educ*, 39, 229–240.

Issenberg, S. B., McGaghie, W. C., Petrusa, E. R., et al. 2005. Features and uses of high-fidelity medical simulations that lead to effective learning: a BEME systematic review. *Med Teach*, 27, 10–28.

Kluger, A. N., DeNisi, A. 1996. The effects of feedback interventions on performance: A historical review, a meta-analysis, and a preliminary feedback intervention theory. *Psychol Bull*, 119, 254–284.

Kruger, J., Dunning, D. 1999. Unskilled and unaware of it: How difficulties in recognizing one's own incompetence lead to inflated self-assessments. *J Pers Soc Psychol*, 77, 1121–1134.

Langebaek, R., Eika, B., Tanggaard, L., et al. 2012. Emotions in veterinary surgical students: A qualitative study. *J Vet Med Educ*, 39, 312–21.

Lefroy, J., Watling, C., Teunissen, P., et al. 2015. Guidelines: the do's, don'ts and don't knows of feedback for clinical education. *Perspect Med Educ*, 4, 284–299.

Luft, J. 1969. *Of Human Interaction.* Palo Alto, CA: National Press Books.

Magnier, K. M., Dale, V. H., Pead, M. J. 2012. Workplace-based assessment instruments in the health sciences. *J Vet Med Educ*, 39, 389–395.

Magnier, K., Pead, M. 2017. Performance and workplace-based assessment. In: *Veterinary Medical Education: A Practical Guide.* Hodgson, J., Pelzer, J. (eds.) Hoboken, NJ: Wiley and Sons, Inc.

Matthew, S. M., Bok, H. G., Chaney, K. P., et al. 2020. Collaborative development of a shared framework for competency-based veterinary education. *J Vet Med Educ*, 47, 578–593.

McGaghie, W. C., Issenberg, S. B., Petrusa, E. R. et al. 2010. A critical review of simulation-based medical education research: 2003-2009. *Med Educ*, 44, 50–63.

Miller, G. 1990. The assessment of clinical skill/competence/ performance. *Acad Med*, 65, 63–67.

Molgaard, L. K., Chaney, K. P., Bok, H. G. J., et al. 2019. Development of core entrustable professional activities linked to a competency-based veterinary education framework. *Med Teach*, 41, 1404–1410.

Molloy, E., Boud, D. 2013. Seeking a different angle on feedback in clinical education: The learner as seeker, judge and user of performance information. *Med Educ*, 47, 227–229.

Mosley, C., Mosley, J. R., Bell, C., et al. 2019. Teaching best practice in hand hygiene: Student use and performance with a gamified gesture recognition system. *Vet Rec*, 185, 444.

Mossop, L., Gray, C., Blaxter, A., et al. 2015. Communication skills training: what the vet schools are doing. *Vet Rec*, 176, 114–117.

Motola, I., Devine, L. A., Chung, H. S., et al. 2013. Simulation in healthcare education: A best evidence practical guide. AMEE Guide No. 82. *Med Teach*, 35, e1511–e1530.

Murdoch-Eaton, D. 2012. Feedback: The complexity of self-perception and the transition from 'transmit' to 'received and understood'. *Med Educ*, 46, 538–540.

Norcini, J. 2005. The mini clinical evaluation exercise (mini-CEX). *Clin Teach*, 2, 25–30.

Norcini, J., Anderson, M. B., Bollela, V., et al. 2018. 2018 consensus framework for good assessment. *Med Teach* 40, 1085–1087.

Norman, G. R., Grierson, L. E., Sherbino, J., et al. 2018. Expertise in medicine and surgery. In: *The Cambridge Handbook of Expertise and Expert Performance*, 2nd Edition. Ericsson, K. A., Hoffman, R. R., Kozbelt, A., et al. (eds.) Cambridge University Press: Cambridge.

Pendleton, D., Scofield, T., Tate, P. et al. 1984. *The Consultation: An Approach to Learning and Teaching*. Oxford: Oxford University Press.

Ramani, S., Krackov, S. K. 2012. Twelve tips for giving feedback effectively in the clinical environment. *Med Teach*, 34, 787–791.

Ramani, S., Konings, K., Mann, K., et al. 2017a. Uncovering the unknown: A grounded theory study exploring the impact of self-awareness on the culture of feedback in residency education. *Med Teach*, 39, 1065–1073.

Ramani, S., Post, S. E., Konings, K., et al. 2017b. "It's just not the culture": A qualitative study exploring residents' perceptions of the impact of institutional culture on feedback. *Teach Learn Med*, 29, 153–161.

Ramani, S., Konings, K. D., Ginsburg, S., et al. 2019a. Meaningful feedback through a sociocultural lens. *Med Teach*, 41, 1342–1352.

Ramani, S., Konings, K. D., Ginsburg, S. et al. 2019b. Twelve tips to promote a feedback culture with a growth mind-set: Swinging the feedback pendulum from recipes to relationships. *Med Teach*, 41, 625–631.

RCVS. 2020. Day One Competences [Online]. RCVS. https://www.rcvs.org.uk/document-library/day-one-competences/ Accessed May 28, 2021.

Read, E. K., Bell, C., Rhind, S., et al. 2015. The use of global rating scales for OSCEs in veterinary medicine. *PLoS One*, 10, e0121000.

Read, E. K., Brown, A., Maxey, C., et al. 2020. Comparing entrustment and competence: An exploratory look at performance-relevant information in the final year of a veterinary program. *J Vet Med Educ*, Advance Online, e20190128.

Rekman, J., Gofton, W., Dudek, N., et al. 2016. Entrustability scales: Outlining their usefulness for competency-based clinical assessment. *Acad Med*, 91, 186–190.

Rich, J. V., Fostaty Young, S., Donnelly, C., et al. 2020. Competency-based education calls for programmatic assessment: But what does this look like in practice? *J Eval Clin Pract*, 26, 1087–1095.

Root Kustritz, M. V. 2017. Pilot study of veterinary student mindset and association with academic performance and perceived stress. *J Vet Med Educ*, 44, 141–146.

Rust, C. 2002. The impact of assessment on student learning: How can the research literature practically help to inform the development of departmental assessment strategies and learner-centred assessment practices? *Act Learn High Educ*, 3, 145–158.

Salisbury, S. K., Chaney, K. P., Ilkiw, J. E., et al. 2019. *Competency- Based Veterinary Education: Part 3 – Milestones*. Washington, DC: AAVMC.

Salisbury, S. K., Rush, B. R., Ilkiw, J. E., et al. 2020. Collaborative development of core entrustable professional activities for veterinary education. *J Vet Med Educ*, 47, 607–618.

Sargeant, J., Mann, K., Sinclair, D., et al. 2008. Understanding the influence of emotions and reflection upon multi-source feedback acceptance and use. *Adv Health Sci Educ Theory Pract*, 13, 275–288.

Sargeant, J. M., Mann, K. V., van der Vleuten, C. P. et al. 2009. Reflection: A link between receiving and using assessment feedback. *Adv Health Sci Educ Theory Pract*, 14, 399–410.

Sargeant, J., Lockyer, J., Mann, K., et al. 2015. Facilitated reflective performance feedback: Developing an evidence- and theory-based model that builds relationship, explores reactions and content, and coaches for performance change (R2C2). *Acad Med*, 90, 1698–1706.

Sargeant, J., Lockyer, J. M., Mann, K., et al. 2018. The R2C2 model in residency education: How does it foster coaching and promote feedback use? *Acad Med*, 93, 1055–1063.

Schuwirth, L. W., van der Vleuten, C. P. 2011. Programmatic assessment: From assessment of learning to assessment for learning. *Med Teach*, 33, 478–485.

Setna, Z., Jha, V., Boursicot, K., et al. 2010. Evaluating the utility of workplace-based assessment tools for speciality training. *Best Pract Res Clin Obstet Gynaecol*, 24, 767–782.

Silverman, J. D., Kurtz, S. M., Draper, J. 1996. The Calgary-Cambridge approach to communication skills teaching 1: Agenda-led, outcome based analysis of the consultation. *Educ Gen Pract*, 4, 288–299.

ten Cate, O., Hart, D., Ankel, F., et al. 2016. Entrustment decision making in clinical training. *Acad Med*, 91, 181–198.

ten Cate, O., Schwartz, A., Chen, H. C. 2020. Assessing trainees and making entrustment decisions: On the nature and use of entrustment-supervision scales. *Acad Med*, 95, 1662–1669.

ten Cate, O., and Taylor, D. R. 2020. The recommended description of an entrustable professional activity: AMEE Guide No. 140. *Med Teach*, Nov 9, 1–9. doi: https://doi.org/10.1080/0142159X.2020.1838465. Epub ahead of print. PMID: 33167763.

Teunissen, P. W., Stapel, D. A., van der Vleuten, C., et al. 2009. Who wants feedback? An investigation of the variables influencing residents' feedback-seeking behavior in relation to night shifts. *Acad Med*, 84, 910–917.

van de Ridder, J. M. M., Stokking, K. M., McGaghie, W., et al. 2008. What is feedback in clinical education? *Med Educ*, 42, 189–197.

van de Ridder, J. M. M., McGaghie, W. C., Stokking, K. M., et al. 2015. Variables that affect the process and outcome of feedback, relevant for medical training: A meta-review. *Med Edcu*, 49, 658–673.

van der Leeuw, R. M., Slootweg, I. A. 2013. Twelve tips for making the best use of feedback. *Med Teach*, 35, 348–351.

van der Vleuten, C. P. 1996. The assessment of professional competence: Developments, research and practical implications. *Adv Health Sci Educ Theory Pract*, 1, 41–67.

van der Vleuten, C. P. M., Schuwirth, L. W. T., Driessen, E. W., et al. 2015. Twelve tips for programmatic assessment. *Med Teach*, 37, 641–646.

van der Vleuten, C., Lindemann, I., Schmidt, L. 2018. Programmatic assessment: The process, rationale and evidence for modern evaluation approaches in medical education. *Med J Aust*, 209, 386–388.

Warman, S., Bell, C., Rhind, S. M. 2014a. Effective student feedback in clinical practice. *In Practice*, 36, 256–258.

Warman, S., Laws, E., Crowther, E., et al. 2014b. Initiatives to improve feedback culture in the final year of a veterinary program. *J Vet Med Educ*, 41, 162–171.

Warman, S. M. 2020. Experiences of recent graduates: Reframing reflection as purposeful, social activity. *Vet Rec*, 186, 347.

Watling, C. J. 2014. Unfulfilled promise, untapped potential: Feedback at the crossroads. *Med Teach*, 36, 692–697.

Watling, C., Driessen, E., van der Vleuten, C. P., et al. 2014. Learning culture and feedback: An international study of medical athletes and musicians. *Med Educ*, 48, 713–723.

Watling, C. J., Ginsburg, S. 2019. Assessment, feedback and the alchemy of learning. *Med Educ*, 53, 76–85.

Weijs, C. A., Coe, J. B., Hecker, K. G. 2015. Final-year students' and clinical instructors' experience of workplace-based assessments used in a small-animal primary-veterinary-care clinical rotation. *J Vet Med Educ*, 42, 382–392.

Whittington, R. E., Rhind, S., Loads, D., et al. 2017. Exploring the link between mindset and psychological well-being among veterinary students. *J Vet Med Educ*, 44, 134–140.

Wilkinson, J., Crossley, J., Wragg, A., et al. 2008. Implementing workplace-based assessments across the medical specialties in the United Kingdom. *Med Educ*, 42, 364–373.

Williamson, J. A., Johnson, J. T., Anderson, S., et al. 2019. A randomized trial comparing freely moving and zonal instruction of veterinary surgical skills using ovariohysterectomy models. *J Vet Med Educ*, 46, 195–204.

6

How Do I Prepare for Assessment and How Do I Know I Am Being Assessed Fairly?

Kate Cobb and Sarah Cripps

School of Veterinary Medicine and Science, University of Nottingham, Sutton Bonington, UK

Introduction

The Objective Structured Clinical Examination (OSCE) has been designed to provide an objective assessment of students' clinical competence and, when implemented effectively, can be part of a robust assessment strategy. To this end, many veterinary schools have incorporated OSCE assessments into their undergraduate curricula (Hardie, 2008). While this enhances assessment of clinical competence, for many students it is a daunting and stressful experience. So how can students best prepare for their OSCE and how can they be assured that they are being subjected to a fair and rigorous assessment of clinical skills? The following chapter will endeavor to address these questions.

Key Messages	
• Assessment can be formative or summative. Be ready to engage with feedback in formative opportunities. • Increasing assessment literacy can increase student confidence and performance during assessments. • Take opportunities to practice clinical skills throughout the course in preparation for assessment. • Identify ways in which you can reduce your own anxiety levels around assessment periods.	• Effective communication with students and all staff involved in the implementation of the OSCE is essential prior to the assessment. • Several methods exist for setting the standard which should be given careful consideration. • Quality assurance measures should be put in place before, during, and after the OSCE assessment.

Psychological Preparation for Exam Performance and Common Barriers to Good Performance

Understanding the Purpose of Assessment

In preparing for any assessment, understanding the purpose of the assessment is important for both the students and assessors. This is often for one or a combination of the following reasons:

- To decide on progression at the end of a phase within a program of study (i.e. does the student advance to the next level?)
- To decide if a student graduates from a program of study
- For selection purposes (e.g. for employment or for entry to more advanced education)
- To provide information to the learner about their development
- As a learning experience
- To provide information to teachers about student progress and performance
- To encourage students to learn

Assessments that generate a grade or have a pass/fail threshold are known as *summative* assessments. These are high-stakes assessments as they are used for progression or graduation purposes and therefore likely to induce higher levels of exam anxiety. Students should be aware of both the consequences of failure in summative assessments and the support available to them should they fail to meet the standard and require remediation. The use of the OSCE in high-stakes summative assessment has become commonplace due to the objective nature of the format and ability to generate reliable and legally defensible scores (Pell et al., 2010).

In contrast, *formative* assessments are used with the intention only to support learning, without a requirement to pass or achieve a certain mark to progress. Assessor feedback on student performance promotes reflective practice and can provide students with the motivation to learn and improve; therefore, formative assessment

opportunities are essential for the development of clinical competence (Ferris and O'Flynn, 2015). Preparation for formative assessment requires a slightly different approach – the assessment is now a diagnostic tool, highlighting areas of strength and weakness and students should be prepared to receive feedback on these areas. For this process to be effective, the learner needs time to understand and reflect on the feedback that is provided to them. An action plan should be created to ensure that feedforward occurs, where targets can be set, and the assessment used to inform and drive future learning.

Consideration needs to be given to the form of the feedback. Verbal feedback often has the advantage of being immediate and promoting a reflective discussion on performance. However, this must be documented in some way for the learner to learn from the assessment. Written feedback is often compiled after the OSCE and, to be most effective, it should be delivered in a timely fashion and be specific to individual performance (Van de Ridder et al., 2008). This has implications for staff resources, and the use of peer-facilitated sessions can be used to reduce the formal staffing requirement. This is discussed later in this chapter (Weyrich et al., 2009).

Educational impact refers to the effect an assessment has on learning behavior. An effective assessment will promote positive student behaviors, improving depth of understanding and practical expertise. Ideally, an OSCE should drive students to develop those skills that they will require during workplace-based learning in clinical years and postgraduation in clinical practice. If the assessment is aligned to appropriate learning outcomes (i.e. clinical competence for a veterinary graduate), a positive educational impact should be achieved.

However, the simulated nature of the OSCE environment and the use of checklists often foster a more strategic approach to assessment. To ensure authenticity, educational impact can be enhanced through consideration of the range and nature of the skills that will be assessed and careful station design. A purely strategic approach should also be discouraged by adopting effective feedback and feedforward strategies in both formative and summative assessments to highlight the importance of skill development to students' future career, rather than "learning to the test."

Increasing Assessment Literacy in Preparation for the OSCE

Assessment literacy refers to an individual's understanding of assessment; specifically, the purpose of the assessment, how it is delivered, and what standard is required for success (Price et al., 2012). It is important that students develop assessment literacy in order to be fully prepared for an OSCE. Table 6.1 describes the elements of assessment literacy, including "the knowledge and understanding of assessment" and "abilities as an examinee and an examiner." It is essential that students have realistic expectations and an appreciation of what the role and limitations of an OSCE are.

One of the aims of an objective assessment is to reduce assessment variation. Simulation is commonplace in OSCE stations to ensure that all students are assessed performing the same tasks the same way. While this may feel less authentic compared to workplace-based assessment for those students who have had the opportunity to practice the same skills in the

Table 6.1 The elements of assessment literacy as described by Price et al. (2012).

Knowledge and understanding of assessment	Abilities as an examinee and an examiner
Appreciation of the assessment's relationship to learning	Skills in self- and peer-assessment
Conceptual understanding of the assessment and its terminology	Understanding of the nature, meaning, and level of assessment criteria and standards
Familiarity with technical approaches to assessment	Ability to select appropriate approaches for relevant assessed tasks

clinic, simulation is key to ensuring a fair assessment for all and reducing the variation inherent in a clinical caseload. To enhance their assessment literacy, students need the opportunity for formative practice and to observe and evaluate a wide range of performance themselves (Rhind and Paterson, 2015).

Practice Is the Key to Success

Preparation for the OSCE will inevitably involve time spent in the clinical skills lab, where students need access to resources to enable them to practice the skills that may be assessed. Practical clinical competence cannot be learnt from a textbook and deliberate practice has been shown to lead to expertise (Duvivier et al., 2011; Ericsson, 2015).

Deliberate practice is more than repetition of a skill or exercise; it involves a structured and focused approach, where feedback is used to inform training and achieve specific goals. Therefore, for practice to be effective, observation of performance and feedback on skills is required. Timetabled formative assessment is an excellent way to provide feedback on learning and skill development; however, opportunities for this structured approach to providing feedback may be limited within the curriculum due to feasibility considerations. Students should therefore be encouraged to seek informal feedback on their performance through practical teaching. This continual "feedback drip" is regularly overlooked by students. Finding time to make routine feedback more explicit and discussing how this can be used to inform future learning can improve student confidence and performance (Lefroy et al., 2015).

OSCE checklists are the individual mark points (items) by which student performance is assessed (Table 6.2 and Appendix 1). These may be made available to students in skills labs to inform their practice and, as a guide, may be helpful to improving performance. However, learners and educators should be mindful of overreliance on this approach. While this may

Table 6.2 Example OSCE checklist for assessment of surgical skills.

Title: Simple interrupted suture pattern

Task	Pass	Fail
Arrives in correct PPE without any prompting		
Places suture square to the incision, 3–5 mm from wound edge		
Ties suture with a square/surgeon's knot		
Single first throw on knots		
Performs correct instrument tie to prevent formation of a granny or running knot		
Places a minimum of 4 throws for a secure knot		
Places simple interrupted sutures to adequately close incision		
Adequate skin edge apposition		
Wound closure tension is appropriate (NO inversion or eversion)		
Uses suture/Mayo scissors to cut suture material		
Trims suture ends to 5–10 mm		
Holds ringed instruments with tripod grip at all times when in use		
Uses forceps (held correctly) to grasp skin		
Ensures knots are to one side of wound		
Maintains surgical sterility		
Overall impression		
Bad fail Fail Borderline Pass Good pass		

Assessors are required to mark each point as either PASS or FAIL; however, weighting may be applied in calculation of the final mark. A global rating scale is included, and assessors are asked to provide their overall impression of the candidate's performance. These judgments can be used to set the threshold passing standard or pass mark of the OSCE station.

improve assessment literacy, students should be encouraged to focus on learning how to perform the complete skill rather than focusing solely on the checklist items. This is not helpful to the development of clinical competence – a complex construct requiring a combination of knowledge, skills, attitudes, and behaviors (Fernandez et al., 2012). Rote learning of checklists in a linear fashion may detract from the depth of thought and problem-based approach required in clinical practice. In short, when considering clinical skills, the sum of the parts may not equal the whole!

Dealing with Exam Anxiety

Assessment is reported as being one of the highest-ranking stressors among students in higher education. Practical examinations, such as the OSCE, have been found to be particularly stressful (Marshall and Jones, 2003; Brand and Schoonheim-Klein, 2009). Veterinary students are often referred to as "high achieving" with "perfectionist traits" and, for such students, pressures may be increased due to fear of failing (Oxtoby, 2018). In addition, many will not have had the experience of having to perform practical skills under direct observation as part of their assessments prior to starting vet school. The OSCE, therefore, is a potentially stressful experience with high levels of exam anxiety, which is not beneficial to mental well-being and does not appear to enhance performance (Brand and Schoonheim-Klein, 2009; Martin and Naziruddin, 2020). Support via tutors and the wider university system should be provided to help students identify ways of dealing with their own anxieties around assessment periods.

It is beyond the scope of this chapter to provide specific advice on dealing with exam anxiety, and a wealth of literature is available on this topic from healthcare providers, self-help books, and the student support services available at individual higher education institutions (Dorland, 2011). It is essential therefore that students are signposted to appropriate sources of support and advice from the start of, and throughout, their veterinary education. However, general guidance for reducing exam anxiety applies to OSCE assessments and the following tips may be helpful:

- Look after your physical self: eat well and take sufficient breaks in the time leading up to the OSCE.
- Continual practice: clinical skills cannot be learnt the night before an exam. It is essential to perform a self-audit and plan the development of your clinical skills throughout the course.
- Be prepared: it is essential to know exactly what will happen on OSCE day.
- Know what works for you: there are many strategies aimed at reducing exam stress, including mindfulness, peer support, and physical exercise. It is important to find out what works for you.

Essential Information for Student Preparation

In addition to the traditional understanding of assessment literacy, it is also important to understand the logistics of the OSCE in the context of each institution and how it is delivered within the clinical skills course. The use of resources that focus on the process rather than the skill (e.g. demonstrating a mock OSCE station that is based around performing an everyday task such as making a cup of tea or a sandwich) can help students with this (Bristol Vet School Clinical Skills Lab, 2020).

Students must be given sufficient information to allow them to prepare properly for the OSCE assessment. They should be informed of the logistical arrangements of the day of the exam, including location and time of assessment, any Personal Protective Equipment requirements, the number of stations they are required to complete, the length of each station, and any "must-pass" elements. OSCE stations can be released to students prior to the exam, which can help to reduce exam anxiety and allows a more focused revision strategy. However, if done too early, this can result in students focusing on assessed skills rather than adopting a more broad and holistic approach to development of their clinical competence. Students should, however, be informed of the types of skill to be assessed, for example whether tasks focus on the psychomotor skill or will other skills be assessed such as communication, teamwork, and professional skills. An example blueprint (Table 6.3) can be shared to allow students to see the types of skills they will be assessed on.

Enhancing Assessment Literacy Through Peer and Self-Assessment

To be fully assessment literate, students need to develop an understanding of the standard that is expected of them and what is required for success. Integration of assessment literacy initiatives within the taught curriculum enables this (Rhind and Paterson, 2015). For OSCE assessments, students can use the opportunity to develop awareness of the expected level of skill performance, compare their own performance and that of their peers to this standard, and understand what constitutes success.

In addition to improving assessment literacy, peer assessment has been shown to reduce

Table 6.3 Example blueprint for a 12-station clinical skills OSCE.

	Clinical exam	Anesthesia and surgery	Laboratory skills	Diagnostic skills	Professional practice
Neurology	Neurological exam of the dog	Abaxial sesamoid nerve block			
Cardiorespiratory		Placing an ET tube			History-taking: coughing dog
Gastrointestinal	Horse with abdominal pain			Lateral abdominal radiograph	
Urinary			Urinalysis	Cystocentesis	
Musculoskeletal			Preparing a smear of joint fluid	Ultrasound of the equine distal limb	
Dermatology	Microscopy: skin scraping	Sub-cutaneous injection			
Reproduction	Bovine rectal exam				Giving information: post-neuter care

Skills are categorized into 5 skill areas and mapped by body system or discipline. The blueprint can be used as evidence of content validity for the OSCE.

exam anxiety, improve student confidence, help guide revision strategy, and improve OSCE performance (Weyrich et al., 2009; Bevan et al., 2019). In addition to assessing their peers, providing the opportunity to participate in OSCE station design and playing the role of the patient have also been shown to be beneficial to learning within medical education (Young et al., 2014; Lee et al., 2018). Peer-assessed OSCEs can therefore be student run and provide a good alternative to formative OSCE assessments that are costly in terms of staff resources and often not feasible to run within the formal curriculum.

Self-assessment forms an integral part of clinical competence, and recognizing limitations is key to the self-regulatory needs of the profession. This can be used alongside peer assessment in preparation for the OSCE (e.g.

reviewing one's own video performance can be useful exam preparation). Improvements in performance not only occur following deliberate practice but also as a result of self-reflection. Self-assessment of video material was found to improve performance among medical students at reassessment following failure. This strategy is likely to be of benefit to those preparing to sit the OSCE at the first attempt, as well as part of a remediation strategy for failing students (White et al., 2009). By allowing students to compare their own clinical skills to the OSCE assessment criteria, their understanding of the expected standards and their own strengths and weaknesses are enhanced. Exemplar video material demonstrating excellent performance may also be helpful in developing a deeper understanding of exactly what is required of the task (Table 6.4).

Table 6.4 Tips for students preparing for an OSCE

Ensuring success: how to be prepared	Barriers to success: what not to do!
Engage with practical skills teaching and formative opportunities throughout the course	Ignore information telling you how the OSCE will run
Construct an action plan for the development of your own clinical skills	Leave practicing skills until the last minute
Utilize your clinical skills center	Arrive unprepared without necessary equipment and PPE
Initiate and engage in opportunities (if available) for peer-assessed OSCEs	Let exam anxiety levels become unmanageable
Read all information provided regarding the OSCE in advance	Rush into the station without considering all the information provided
Know where you need to be and when	
Ensure you have all the essential equipment and PPE to complete the OSCE	

Standard Setting Techniques – What Are They, Principles of How They Work and Are Applied

What Is the Standard?

Pass/fail decisions on an OSCE should be made using predetermined criteria against which the student is evaluated, allowing for transparency in setting expectations and helping to provide feedback on performance. This chapter provides a general overview of standard setting techniques. McKinley and Norcini (2014) and Pell (2010) provide further information on the principles of standard setting and how these are applied to the OSCE in healthcare education.

The "standard" refers to the score required to be successful in the OSCE assessment. This is usually derived from an average or the sum of the scores required to pass each individual station, known as the *station standard* (Wass et al., 2001). When considering clinical competence, it might be considered inappropriate to allow compensation between different types of skills. For this reason, in addition to achieving the standard score, passing a minimum number of stations is usually required to pass an OSCE assessment. In some institutions, critical stations

are identified, which must be passed for the candidate to be successful. For example, a student could perform poorly on a station requiring emergency care and cardiopulmonary resuscitation but pass the OSCE based on performance in other skills and disciplines if compensation between stations is allowed. If emergency care is considered a critical skill at this stage, students could be required to pass that station for progression. However, the reliability of one station is insufficient to make high stakes decision; therefore, failing students must be given the opportunity to repeat any must-pass elements.

Defining the standard is complex and can be challenging. What does competent performance look like? Perhaps more importantly, what constitutes incompetence and failure to achieve a pass on a station? These questions are not easily answered and can lead to much debate between assessors. To understand how the standard is set, we first need to explore ways of scoring students within the station.

Marking Criteria: Checklists or Global Rating Scales

OSCE stations can be scored using either a global rating scale (GRS), a checklist, or a combination of both. A GRS requires assessors to compare students to the expected performance of a student at the same stage of the course and make a judgment based on overall performance, often encompassing several domains of clinical competence. Use of a GRS is often viewed as being a more holistic method of assessment, but it requires expert assessors and may be more appropriate for more advanced students in later stages of the veterinary course (Read and Bell 2015). Conversely, a checklist breaks the skill down into component parts, each with a binary response (i.e. *yes* or *no*, *pass* or *fail*). Checklists do not necessarily require expert assessors and may be better suited to the early years where a more structured approach to clinical and practical skills is adopted.

Both checklists and global rating scales can be used in combination for comparison of the two methods and to set the standard (Table 6.2). Both methods have been shown to have acceptable levels of reliability (Read et al., 2015); however, concerns have been raised that, as expertise increases, the person being assessed may be at a disadvantage if checklists alone are used. This is because when experts perform a skill, they may not demonstrate certain steps on the checklist. As such, the assessment may fail to capture an expert's proficiency (even though the expert clearly knows what they are doing. . .), and they may end up scoring the same or even lower than less-experienced students who demonstrated each individual step on the checklist (Hodges et al., 1999).

Methods of Calculating the Standard

Whether checklists or global rating scales are used, a decision needs to be made on how the standard score will be derived. Several methods have been described within the literature and are described below:

Angoff method: Prior to the examination, a panel of standard setters considers what percentage of "borderline candidates" would achieve the minimum standard on each station.

The borderline candidate is a student who neither clearly passes nor fails the station – their performance is around the pass mark. Consideration needs to be given to the makeup of the panel and who is best placed to make those decisions for the stage of the veterinary program. Panel members should include experts within the disciplines being assessed and those involved in teaching the practical skills who have an insight into the students' capabilities and the skill level of a borderline student. Discussion of the borderline student and the minimum expected standard among panel members is important when using this approach.

Once the panel has reached a decision on the percentage of borderline students expected to pass each station, these numbers are averaged to produce the pass mark for the OSCE exam as a whole (Ben-David, 2000; McKinley and Norcini, 2014). Table 6.5 provides an example of how Angoff's method can be used to arrive at the standard for a five-station OSCE using a panel of 10 standard setters. Several modifications to the Angoff method described above have been proposed and evaluated in different educational settings (Hurtz and Auerbach, 2003). Despite modification, the Angoff method can be time consuming, requiring meetings of panel members prior to the assessment to set the standard. Alternative methods, such as the overlapping groups and borderline regression methods, discussed below, utilize judgments made during the assessment and may be more feasible for many programs.

Overlapping groups: In contrast to the Angoff method, in the "overlapping groups" method, the standard is set based on examinee performance. The assessors complete both a checklist and make a global judgment on a candidate as *pass* or *fail*. The scores of passing and failing students are plotted separately (Figure 6.1). In this case, the standard is usually the point at which the lines intersect; however, it can be adjusted to minimize false positives (e.g. in high-stakes exams where passing students are then given increasing clinical responsibility) (Downing et al., 2006).

Table 6.5 Angoff method to calculate the standard on a five-station OSCE.

Station	Standard setter										Mean average
	1	2	3	4	5	6	7	8	9	10	
1	60	75	50	65	50	50	70	55	60	55	59.0
2	75	80	55	70	75	70	75	65	80	70	71.5
3	60	65	55	60	65	60	65	50	60	60	60.0
4	70	75	60	75	65	80	75	75	70	60	70.5
5	65	65	50	60	55	50	55	60	65	65	59.0
Standard											**320**

Each of the ten standard setters estimate the percentage of borderline students who would achieve the minimum standard at each of the five stations. The mean average provides the standard required to pass each station. These station standards are summed to provide the OSCE standard. In the example shown, a score of 320 would be required to pass the OSCE.

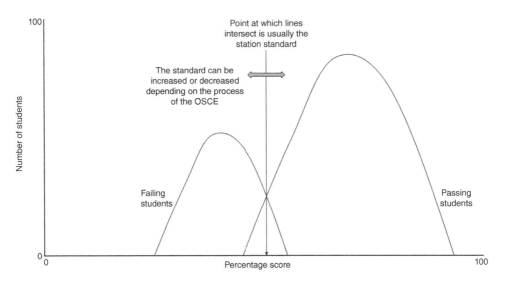

Figure 6.1 The "overlapping groups" method can be used to determine the station standard as a percentage score for 100 students. For high-stakes exams, the intersect is moved to the right to minimize false positives. In lower-stakes exams (e.g. where the purpose is more formative), the intersect can be moved to the left to reduce the number of false negatives.

Likewise, for lower-stakes assessments with a more formative focus, the standard can be adjusted to minimize false negatives and the number of failing students.

Borderline group: Similar to the overlapping groups method, when using the "borderline group" method, assessors complete a checklist and also make a judgment using a three-point global scale: "pass," "fail," or "borderline." Next, the scores of borderline candidates are considered for each station. Their checklist scores are averaged, and this value becomes the pass score for that station. Each station score is then either summed or averaged to get the pass score for the entire examination – "the standard" (McKinley and Norcini, 2014). This method can be problematic when dealing with small cohorts since the standard for the entire group is essentially being set based on the performance of a few candidates who have been identified as being borderline.

Borderline regression: This method also requires assessors to complete both a checklist and a global rating scale. Regression analysis is then performed using the global rating scores as the independent variable and the checklist scores as the dependent variable. The equation and graph produced are used to find the pass score, usually set at or just above the borderline group (Figure 6.2). This method has the advantage of using evaluations of all examinees in the cohort to set the standard (Wood et al., 2006). It should be noted that in cohorts of less than 50, which may be encountered in the context of reassessment, standard setting methods that rely on examinee performance, including borderline regression, become unreliable.

Compromise methods have been described such as the Hofstee (McKinley and Norcini, 2014), in which standard setters make judgments regarding the number of students passing and failing, as well as the minimum and maximum acceptable standard score. However, the use of relative judgments makes these less suitable for summative assessments. Lastly, Ebel weighting has also been used for OSCE standard setting with smaller cohorts but is less common, having been primarily developed for knowledge-related tests (Violato et al., 2003).

Quality Assurance in OSCEs – Reasons Why Stations and Learners Exhibit Variability

While the OSCE has been developed to ensure a fair test of all examinees, variation still occurs within stations. Quality assurance measures are utilized to identify and minimize sources of variation, which can include individual assessors, simulated clients, live animals, equipment and resources, and student performance. Two key terms in considering quality assurance are *validity* and *reliability*. Validity can be described as a measurement of how well an OSCE assesses what it

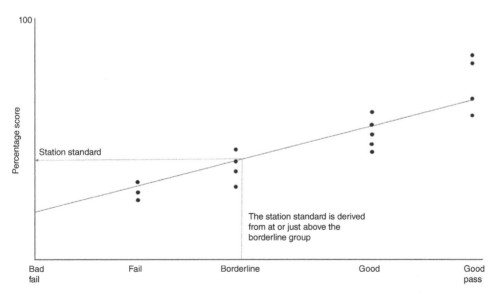

Figure 6.2 The borderline regression method to calculate the station standard. The graph illustrates how checklist scores (black dots) are plotted against the global ratings. The regression line is used to determine the station standard, shown by the gray arrow.

is intended to assess, while reliability refers to the consistency or repeatability of the results.

Validity

Traditionally, validity had been described as having several different component parts (Table 6.6). However, validity is more recently considered to be a singular entity that also incorporates reliability, since no assessment can be valid if it is not reliable (Messick, 1992; Downing, 2003).

To ensure *content validity*, an exam blueprint should be created as part of the OSCE development. A blueprint allows the stations within the OSCE to be mapped to course outcomes, topics, skill areas, and species. While it is not feasible to assess all skills in all species areas, it is important that a representative sample of skills is assessed. A blueprint provides evidence of this (Table 6.3).

Content validity provides evidence of curriculum alignment, whereby the assessment is aligned to what is taught and the way in which it is delivered. Part of the quality assurance process should consider curriculum alignment, including the way that students are asked to perform a task and the criteria that are used to assess them during the OSCE (which must reflect how the skills are taught within a course). This is particu-

larly important when the assessors are not involved in curriculum design and teaching.

Content validity is important when considering case specificity, a recognized phenomenon in clinical education. First described by Elstein et al. (1978), case specificity states that problem-solving and clinical performance will vary between cases, even among experts. Applying this to the OSCE, we can assume that even the high achieving students will have "bad cases" where their performance may be less than satisfactory. Therefore, to gain a reliable impression of student competence, an OSCE requires a sufficient number of stations to allow for this variation in performance in order to produce an outcome that is representative of an individual's abilities.

Factors impacting validity should be considered prior to the assessment. For example, is the method of scoring a student appropriate for the skills being assessed? Some complex constructs such as communication, proficiency, and professionalism do not lend themselves to assessment using a checklist, so use of global rating scales and expert assessors are likely to result in enhanced *construct validity* in these situations. OSCE stations in veterinary medicine are traditionally five minutes long; however, this may not be sufficient to complete some tasks, particularly in the later stages of

Table 6.6 Traditional components of validity.

Type	Definition
Face	The extent to which a test appears practical, pertinent, and related to its purpose (Mosier, 1947)
Content	The adequacy with which the instrument samples the domain of measurement (Hecker and Violato, 2009)
Criterion	A comparison of test scores with one or more external variables (criteria) considered to provide a direct measure of the characteristic or behavior in question (Messick, 1992)
Predictive	The certainty to which a test can predict future performance (Dent et al., 2017)
Concurrent	The degree to which scores on a test correlate with the scores on an established test administered at the same time (Dent et al., 2017)
Construct	The measurement of some attribute or quality, which is not operationally defined (Cronbach and Meehl, 1955)

the course where multiple domains are being assessed. The validity of the assessment will be compromised if the task cannot be performed in the time available; therefore, realistic trialing of each station prior to running the assessment is essential to ensure the task is achievable.

Authenticity is an important consideration in an OSCE assessment, particularly when used in the clinical phases of veterinary education. Students who have been exposed to clinical practice and have had opportunities to develop their competence in the workplace may challenge the validity of assessment in a simulated environment. Care should be taken to ensure that, when used, simulated clients and resources represent the clinical workplace as closely as possible (i.e. to enhance *face validity*).

Reliability

Despite being labeled an "objective" assessment, this does not always assure reliability. A poorly designed OSCE can have low reliability. Likewise, some observational judgments include a degree of subjectivity, which can lead to variation in scores and low reliability. The OSCE is generally considered to be a robust and reliable assessment of clinical skills (hence, its use in summative assessments); however, this cannot be automatically assumed, and evaluating the reliability of an OSCE assessment should always be part of the quality assurance process.

Psychometric tests such as the *KR20* and *Cronbach's alpha* are commonly used as measures of reliability. Strictly speaking, these are measures of internal consistency, not reliability; however these terms are often used interchangeably. Alpha values of greater than 0.7 are generally considered acceptable for summative assessment purposes. While these measures provide information about the internal consistency of the test, they do not give any indication of the source of error when reliability is poor. Generalizability theory can be used in this instance to determine the sources of variation within an OSCE (Tavakol and Dennick, 2012). In an ideal assessment, the only source of

variation would come from the difference in students' ability to perform the tasks; however, in reality, multiple sources of potential variation exist. Generalizability theory is particularly helpful where OSCEs take place, for example, over different sites, days, and/or with different assessors since it enables the greatest sources of variation within the scores to be identified.

When developing the OSCE, several factors should be considered, which can improve the reliability of the assessment. It is important to pilot the individual stations to ensure the skills can be performed in the time available. Clarity of marking criteria will reduce variation between assessors, known as *inter-rater reliability*. Assessors should be thoroughly familiar with the content of the station and the marking criteria. Therefore, assessor training is required to ensure adequate inter-rater reliability. Where multiple versions of the same station are run, a lead assessor can be assigned, who has been involved in the teaching and assessment design. Their role is to provide appropriate briefing/training and guidance for the team of assessors assigned to that station, improving both reliability and curricular alignment. In addition to reducing the effect of case specificity and enhancing content validity, increasing the number of observations will also result in increasing the reliability of the assessment. Adequate reliability can be achieved with between 14 and 18 stations; however, feasibility must be considered when deciding on the length of the OSCE (Epstein, 2007). More stations and increased testing time generally result in increased reliability, but there comes a point where adding more stations is logistically impossible and the assessment burden to both staff and students must be considered. More recently, 10–12 stations have been suggested as an ideal compromise likely to result in acceptable reliability, but this comes with a note of caution as 12 poorly designed stations may result in lower reliability than 8 well-designed OSCE stations (Dent et al., 2017).

In addition to validity and reliability, quality assurance measures should also consider other elements of assessment utility – namely, feasibility, acceptability, and educational impact (van der Vleuten, 1996). The feasibility of running an OSCE assessment frequently results in a compromise on the numbers and design of stations. Acceptability to both staff and students is essential and will also influence the OSCE design and implementation. Finally, a good OSCE will engage students and have a positive impact on their approaches to learning and development of their clinical competence.

Post-Exam Analysis

While it is desirable to develop a robust OSCE prior to exam delivery, post-examination analysis is essential to the overall quality assurance process. The results need to be credible – for example too few or all students passing may not be acceptable to the context. Measures of reliability and validity are used for post-exam analysis to identify sources of variation and to ensure that the results represent a fair assessment of the students' abilities. Concerns raised by students and assessors either during or immediately after the OSCE should also be considered as part of this process. Individual station standards should be reviewed, and moderation may be required where inconsistency may have resulted in one or more groups of students being at a disadvantage. Moderation might involve adjustment of marks for a particular group or removal of an entire station. In addition to informing any moderation of results, post-exam analysis should be used to improve future examinations. For example, individual assessor performance can be used to promote discussion around standards and expectations so as to minimize future inter-rater variation. Lessons can be learnt regarding station design, checklist items, and instructions to both students and assessors.

It is important for each program to develop its own quality assurance process. An example quality assurance checklist is shown in Table 6.7, which may help schools and individuals in preparing for, and ensuring the quality of, the OSCE assessment. Further detail on the development and implementation of an OSCE has been previously described (Davis et al., 2006, Khan et al., 2013).

How Does Assessment in the Workplace Differ from That in the Skills Center?

The OSCE has been adopted by many veterinary schools due to the perceived robustness of assessment through reduced variation of assessed tasks and objective checklists resulting in a fair assessment of all students. However, there is a compromise in validity when compared to assessment of skill and case management in the clinical workplace. While assessment of competence through an OSCE tells us what an individual is *capable of doing*, performance or workplace-based assessment relates to what an individual *actually does* in everyday practice (Miller, 1990). Unlike an OSCE where each student completes the same tasks and is assessed using the same grading schemes, there is variation in workplace-based assessment relating to the nature and complexity of the tasks, the temperaments of patients, potential client involvement, the clinic itself, and staff relationships. Assessors bring an additional source of variation. They are often performing the roles of teacher, supervisor, clinician, and assessor simultaneously; therefore, this, along with the complexities of the clinic, can influence the way in which students are evaluated. Any single observation in the clinic is therefore inherently unreliable, so it is important that workplace-based assessment consists of a series of observations that are used collectively to make any high-stakes decisions regarding clinical competence.

Multiple tools have been developed for assessment in the workplace including the mini-clinical evaluation exercise (Mini-CEX), direct observation of procedural skills (DOPS), multi-source feedback or $360°$ assessment, and case-based discussions (CbD) (Hecker et al., 2012). While it is beyond the scope of this chapter to describe each of these assessment tools in detail,

Table 6.7 Quality assurance checklist.

Selecting stations	• Identify potential stations to assess • Create OSCE blueprint • Check feasibility of space and resources
Station development	• Ensure input from teaching faculty during station writing • Development of instructions for candidates, examiners, technical support staff, and simulated clients • Internal review of stations • Review of all stations by external examiners • Trial stations • Agree on standard setting method
Communication	• Training of assessors • Training of simulated patients and/or clients • Release of station information to students • Notify students of formative practice opportunities
Running the OSCE	• Station set up including any audio and IT support requirements prior to the day of assessment • Briefing of candidates and assessors on the day • Note any concerns from assessors or students during the OSCE
Post-examination review	• Post-exam analysis regarding reliability of stations • Check that percentage of students passing and failing is acceptable to context • Investigate any student and assessor concerns • Moderation of marks, including removal of stations if deemed necessary
Feedback	• Feedback to students on performance • Notify students of any reassessment requirements • Notify students of remediation opportunities • Feedback to assessors on performance • Feedback from assessors for station improvement

it should be emphasized that implementation and interpretation of scores are more important to effective workplace-based assessment than the tool itself (See Chapter 6 for further details).

Often, due to time or resource constraints, the OSCE provides assessment of part of a task, providing a snapshot into clinical competence. There is more opportunity in workplace-based assessment for the complete task to be assessed, including skills such as teamwork and professional attitude and behavior. Hence, workplace-based assessment is frequently seen as a more valid and authentic assessment of clinical competence.

The main purpose of workplace-based assessment should be to provide feedback on performance and an opportunity to discuss and plan future learning. Given the multiple observations required if any summative judgments are to be made, this can prove challenging logistically. Making the time and finding space within a busy clinic to deliver meaningful individual feedback can be problematic. Care should be taken that the purpose of the assessment is maintained, and a program of workplace-based assessment does not evolve into a hoop-jumping exercise, where checklists are signed, but feedback is forgotten.

Workplace-based assessment provides a natural progression from the OSCE and has advantages in its authenticity and validity; however, challenges exist regarding feasibility and reliability of individual observations. To be a true assessment of what a student *does*, observation and assessment should be opportunistic, without emphasis on preparation for assessment. However, we may never achieve a true assessment of what a student "does" in practice in the undergraduate curriculum, because as soon as a patient encounter is defined as an assessment opportunity, the student's behavior changes and they may revert to the "shows how" of the task being done, rather than what they "do" in everyday practice.

References

Ben-David, M. F. 2000. AMEE Guide No. 18: Standard setting in student assessment. *Med Teach*, 22, 120–130.

Bevan, J., Russell, B., Marshall, B. 2019. A new approach to OSCE preparation-PrOSCEs. *BMC Med Educ*, 19, 126.

Brand, H., Schoonheim-Klein, M. 2009. Is the OSCE more stressful? Examination anxiety and its consequences in different assessment methods in dental education. *Eur J Dent Educ*, 13, 147–153.

Bristol Vet School Clinical Skills Lab. 2020. OSCE Guide https://www.youtube.com/watch?v=5mP4Jmxf9mc&feature=youtu.be Accessed September 27, 2020.

Cronbach, L. J., Meehl, P. E. 1955. Construct validity in psychological tests. *Psychol Bull*, 52, 281–302.

Davis, M. H., Ponnamperuma, G. G., McAleer, S., et al. 2006. The Objective Structured Clinical Examination (OSCE) as a determinant of veterinary clinical skills. *J Vet Med Educ*, 33, 578–587.

Dent, J. A., Harden, R. M., Hunt, D., et al. 2017. *A Practical Guide for Medical Teachers*, 5th Edition. New York, NY: Elsevier.

Dorland, S. 2011. *Exam Stress?: No Worries!*. Hoboken, USA: John Wiley & Sons.

Downing, S. M. 2003. Validity: On the meaningful interpretation of assessment data. *Med Educ*, 37, 830–837.

Downing, S. M., Tekian, A., Yudkowsky, R. 2006. Procedures for establishing defensible absolute passing scores on performance examinations in health professions education. *Teach Learn Med*, 18, 50–57.

Duvivier, R. J., van Dalen, J., Muijtjens, A. M., et al. 2011. The role of deliberate practice in the acquisition of clinical skills. *BMC Med Educ*, 11, 101.

Elstein, A. S., Shulman, L. S., Sprafka, S. A. 1978. *Medical Problem Solving: An Analysis of Clinical Reasoning*. Cambridge, Massachusetts: Harvard University Press.

Epstein, R. M. 2007. Assessment in medical education. *N Engl J Med*, 356, 387–396.

Ericsson, K. A. 2015. Acquisition and maintenance of medical expertise: A perspective from the expert-performance approach with deliberate practice. *Acad Med*, 90, 1471–1486.

Fernandez, N., Dory, V., Ste-Marie, L. G., et al. 2012. Varying conceptions of competence: an analysis of how health sciences educators define competence. *Med Educ*, 46, 357–365.

Ferris, H., O'Flynn, D. 2015. Assessment in medical education; What are we trying to achieve? *Int J High Educ*, 4, 139–144.

Hardie, E. M. 2008. Current methods in use for assessing clinical competencies: what works? *J Vet Med Educ*, 35, 359–368.

Hecker, K. G., Norris, J., Coe, J. B. 2012. Workplace-based assessment in a primary-care setting. *J Vet Med Educ*, 39, 229–240.

Hecker K., Violato C. 2009. Validity, reliability, and defensibility of assessments in veterinary education. *J Vet Med Educ*, 36, 271–275.

Hodges, B., McNaughton, N., Tiberius, R. 1999. OSCE checklists do not capture increasing levels of expertise. *Acad Med*, 74, 1129–1134.

Hurtz, G. M., Auerbach, M. A. 2003. A meta-analysis of the effects of modifications to the

Angoff method on cutoff scores and judgment consensus. *Educ Psychol Meas*, *63*, 584–601.

Khan, K. Z., Gaunt, K., Ramachandran, S., et al. 2013. The objective structured clinical examination (OSCE): AMEE guide no. 81. part II: Organisation & administration. *Med Teach*, 35, e1447–e1463.

Lee, C. B., Madrazo, L., Khan, U., et al. 2018. A student-initiated objective structured clinical examination as a sustainable cost-effective learning experience. *Med Educ Online*, 23, 1440111.

Lefroy, J., Watling, C., Teunissen, P. W, et al. 2015. Guidelines: The do's, don'ts and don't knows of feedback for clinical education. *Perspect Med Educ*, 4, 284–299.

Marshall, G., Jones, N. 2003. A pilot study into the anxiety induced by various assessment methods. *Radiography*, 9, 185–191.

Martin, R.D., Naziruddin, Z. 2020. Systematic review of student anxiety and performance during objective structured clinical examinations. *Curr Pharm Teach Learn*, 12, 1491–1497.

McKinley, D. W., Norcini, J. J. 2014. How to set standards on performance-based examinations: AMEE Guide No. 85. *Med Teach*, 36, 97–110.

Messick, S. 1992. Validity of test interpretation and use. In: *Encyclopedia of Educational Research*, 6th Edition. Alkin, M. C. (ed.) New York: MacMillan.

Miller, G. E. 1990. The assessment of clinical skills/competence/performance. *Acad Med*, 65, S63–S67.

Mosier, C. I. 1947. A critical examination of the concepts of face validity. *Educ Psychol Meas*, 7, 191–205.

Oxtoby, C. 2018. Managing perfectionism. *Vet Rec*, 183, 106.

Pell, G., Fuller, R., Homer, M., et al. 2010. How to measure the quality of the OSCE: A review of metrics–AMEE guide no. 49. *Med Teach*, 32, 802–811.

Price, M., Rust, C., O'Donovan, B., et al. 2012. *Assessment Literacy: The Foundation for Improving Student Learning*. Wheatley, UK: Oxford Centre for Staff and Learning Development, Oxford Brookes University.

Read, E. K., Bell, C., Rhind, S., et al. 2015. The use of global rating scales for OSCEs in veterinary medicine. *PLoS One*, 10, e0121000.

Rhind, S. M., Paterson, J. 2015. Assessment literacy: Definition, implementation, and implications. *J Vet Med Educ*, 42, 28–35.

Tavakol, M., Dennick, R. 2012. Post-examination interpretation of objective test data: monitoring and improving the quality of high-stakes examinations: AMEE Guide No. 66. *Med Teach*, 34, e161–e175.

Van de Ridder, J. M., Stokking, K. M., McGaghie, W. C., et al. 2008. What is feedback in clinical education? *Med Educ*, 42, 189–197.

van der Vleuten, C. P. 1996. The assessment of professional competence: Developments, research and practical implications. *Adv Health Sci Eeuc Theory Pract*, 1, 41–67.

Violato, C., Marini, A., Lee, C. 2003. A validity study of expert judgement procedures for setting cut-off scores on high-stakes credentialling examinations using cluster analysis. *Eval Health Prof*, 26, 59–72.

Wass, V., van der Vleuten, C., Shatzer, J., et al. 2001. Assessment of clinical competence. *Lancet*, 357, 945–949.

Weyrich, P., Celebi, N., Schrauth, M., et al. 2009. Peer-assisted versus faculty staff-led skills laboratory training: A randomised controlled trial. *Med Eeuc*, 43, 113–120.

White, C. B., Ross, P. T., Gruppen, L. D. 2009. Remediating students' failed OSCE performances at one school: The effects of self-assessment, reflection, and feedback. *Acad Med*, 84, 651–654.

Wood, T. J., Humphrey-Murto, S. M., Norman, G. R. 2006. Standard setting in a small scale OSCE: A comparison of the modified borderline-group method and the borderline regression method. *Adv Health Sci Educ Theory Pract*, 11, 115–122.

Young, I., Montgomery, K., Kearns, P., et al. 2014. The benefits of a peer-assisted mock OSCE. *Clin Teach*, 11, 214–218.

7

How Can I Best Learn in a Simulated Environment?

Julie A. Hunt, Stacy L. Anderson, and Jennifer T. Johnson

College of Veterinary Medicine, Lincoln Memorial University, Harrogate, TN, USA

Box 7.1 Key Messages

- Students learn clinical skills through deliberate practice with specific feedback on how to improve their performance
- Live animals offer the highest degree of realism but they can be harmed by students during practice, they can injure students, they can trigger anxiety, and they require husbandry and care. Use of live animals for practice can also raise ethical issues

- Although cadaver tissue is more difficult to source, handle and dispose of, there are some teaching settings where it is useful
- Despite variation in fidelity or realism, models have much to offer: safety, standardization, and repetitive practice
- Comprehensive clinical skills programs use live animals, cadavers and models in varying capacities to meet teaching and assessment needs

---

How Are Skills Taught?

Historically, clinical skills have been taught using an apprenticeship model – the "see one, do one, teach one" paradigm of surgical training that was made mainstream by William Stewart Halsted over a century ago (Halsted, 1904). His method of training surgery residents was adapted to training veterinary surgeons and remains a common training method, although it is increasingly being replaced by training in a clinical skills laboratory.

Training in a clinical skills laboratory is more controlled, safer, can be standardized, and graduated levels of complexity may be added to allow learners to progressively develop and demonstrate their skills. Learners may be taught using a combination of models, cadavers, and live animals in order to meet predetermined learning objectives. Since a comprehensive clinical skills curriculum is not dependent on access to clinical cases that require specific procedures to be performed, students' training and educational outcomes are more consistent than with traditional clinical training alone.

How Are Skills Learned?

The development of expert performance in medicine and surgery depends on deliberate practice – the pursuit of intense, repetitive

---

skills practice with rigorous assessment and specific feedback before advancement to the next level of difficulty (Ericsson, 2004). As clinical skills are taught, practice sessions and planned repetition of tasks are necessary to allow competence to develop. Regular assessment, most frequently low-stakes in nature, is necessary to ensure that students have achieved the desired level of proficiency. On-going timely, specific feedback is critical to guiding students as they grow in competence.

Live Animals

Live animals remain the best option for teaching noninvasive skills that require the highest degree of fidelity or realism (Figure 7.1). No model or simulator will ever be as realistic. For this reason, live animal training is typically readily accepted by students and faculty as helpful to the educational process. However, individual animals do possess variations in temperament, anatomy, and function. For example, horses used in a veterinary teaching program are often extremely docile and may not resemble the horses that a student is likely to encounter while working in a private practice setting with a typical horse population.

Live animals provide real-time feedback to students via their behavior, pain responses, aversion, bleeding, or bruising. Live animals may vocalize, evade capture, or kick or bite if they are unhappy. All of these actions provide feedback to the student that what the student is doing is not well-accepted and the student can learn to alter the way they are treating the animal. Instructor supervision and feedback in these situations is critical to improving student technique, safeguarding animal welfare and preventing student injury while they are practicing their skills. Since live animals can be harmed or suffer pain from inexperienced students, greater student preparation, enhanced emphasis on safety practices, and more supervision are required while students practice their skills on live animals than when cadavers or models are used.

One drawback to utilizing live animals for the practice of invasive procedures, such as performing sterilization surgery, is that the majority of students practicing this task have reported feeling nervous, scared, or worried

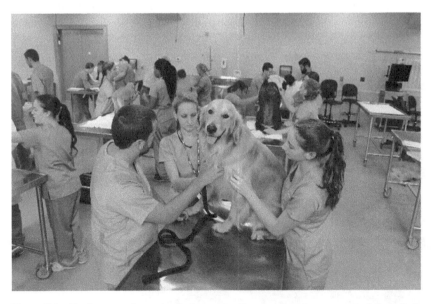

Figure 7.1 Students perform physical examinations on live dogs as part of their first-year clinical skills curriculum.

about inadvertently harming the animal (Langebæk et al., 2012a). These negative emotions can interfere with the learning process and can negatively impact student well-being. However, prior practice with surgical skills models can reduce these negative emotions (Langebæk et al., 2012b).

The use of live animals is further complicated by institutional and national regulations that require written approval for the procurement, care, use, and disposition of animals. Some skills may require rest times in between uses, such as for sedation or phlebotomy. Scheduling laboratory sessions around these required rest periods and limitations on animal use may make achieving deliberate practice challenging for students. Animals are also labor intensive and costly to maintain because they require appropriate food, water, exercise, housing, and daily care. If students are to be involved in the care of the animals, who will supervise the care, and what is the consequence for a student who fails to provide adequate care? Policies must be in place to address issues that inevitably arise with students and live animal care.

Live animals are important for clinical skills training, but with time, their use is likely to become more regulated and ethically limited. Live animals are probably best used for less-invasive procedures, including teaching and practicing animal handling, or for procedures that students have previously received training for using models or cadavers. Later in this chapter, an example will be provided of how to integrate live animal use with models for teaching animal handling to veterinary students over the span of several semesters.

Cadavers

Cadavers and cadaver tissue may seem like a natural alternative to using live animals, and they have several advantages (Figure 7.2). Cadavers cannot be harmed or suffer pain from inexperienced student use, and they don't scratch, bite, or kick. Students can practice a multitude of procedures on a single cadaver, and sometimes fewer institutional approvals are necessary. Cadavers are accepted by students as being realistic learning tools because, although the animal is dead, in most instances they still look reasonably life-like. It is also worth pointing out that this can vary depending on the condition of the cadaver and the length of time since the animal expired, so unlike models that are very standardized in appearance, cadavers tend not to be.

Cadavers also have numerous downsides. Although they may look like live animals, not all

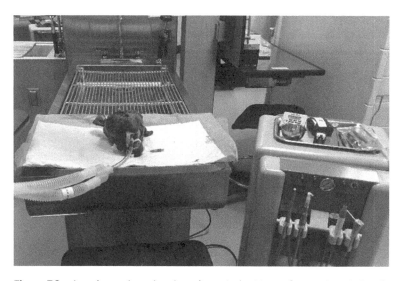

Figure 7.2 A canine cadaver head awaits a student to perform a dental cleaning and extractions.

of their tissues handle or respond like living tissues. From the moment of death, blood no longer runs through vessels and the tissues begin to autolyze. Cadavers often have an unpleasant odor or appearance, although these can be assuaged by partial preservation or soft embalming. If frozen, cadavers may require several days at room temperature or soaking in water baths to fully thaw, which can be inconvenient and unpleasant for personnel and often requires significant space. Cadavers may also pose potential biohazard and/ or chemical risks if they are preserved, and they typically require low temperature storage.

When used in clinical skills laboratories, cadavers do not offer the vital feedback that live animals do (e.g. pain response, bleeding, bruising), so all feedback must be offered by an observer monitoring a student's technique. Because cadaver tissue typically has a short life span and is not left out beyond a single teaching session, it also does not typically offer repetitive practice for continued skills development.

The procurement and use of cadavers can also create special concerns. In some regions, cadavers may be difficult to source, are expensive if purchased, and can raise ethical questions regarding their source. Alternative sources of cadavers include willed body programs and obtaining abattoir material where available. The use of cadavers may place an emotional burden on students, particularly if the cadaver assigned to the student resembles the student's pet at home. Draping the cadavers and allowing students to switch to a different cadaver if theirs look too familiar can be helpful in decreasing that emotional strain.

In short, though they may be helpful in teaching a few targeted skills that models are not able to replicate adequately, cadavers come with a lot of negative qualities. For example, models may not be able to replicate the precise look of certain anatomic structures such as the larynx or the ventral abdominal wall, the anatomy of which are important for endotracheal intubation and celiotomy closure. If students have already practiced these tasks on a low-fidelity model but would benefit from seeing an anatomically accurate model of the relevant structures before performing these skills on a live animal, cadaver tissue may offer a good intermediate solution. Cadavers may also be helpful for teaching emergency procedures that are not amenable to practicing on models due to complexity, such as chest tube thoracostomy.

Models

Models or simulators of all types have become extremely prevalent in clinical skills laboratories worldwide (Figure 7.3). Models are student

Figure 7.3 A student performs a circumferential ligature on an ovariohysterectomy model.

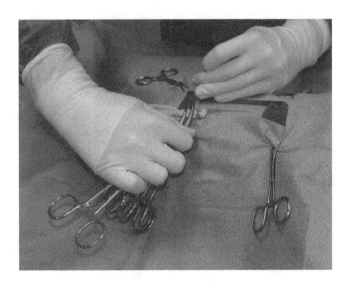

friendly, being able to be used and reused on a student's own time. Some veterinary schools make models available to students in a drop-in skills practice area, while other schools may send certain high-use models home with students. Students working on models require less immediate faculty supervision, as models do not scratch, bite, or kick students. Models do not suffer pain if used incorrectly, though they can potentially be damaged by improper use or extremes in temperature. Models do not typically require special storage, care, or disposal, and they do not present ethical issues related to sourcing.

Models can be standardized so that all students receive the same training or can be assessed on the same task. A series of standardized models with related assessments can be thoughtfully built into a comprehensive clinical skills curriculum, making a student's skills training independent of patient availability. Models may also be able to be adjusted to accommodate a more advanced student through altering certain aspects of the model. Adequate and timely feedback is easier to deliver in a simulated environment where a procedure can be stopped at any time to allow students the opportunity to immediately correct a mistake or repeat a portion of the performance. Models can be used to portray normal or abnormal conditions and can allow students to practice rare emergency procedures that cannot otherwise be practiced.

Models do require storage space, which should be considered when building facilities. Few clinical skills laboratories have ever found themselves with adequate storage space. Some models can be costly, especially the initial purchase price for higher-fidelity models. Budgets should consider the purchase price, the replacement parts, and the on-going maintenance, possible warranty costs, and eventual replacement of the models, as all models do inevitably have a finite life span, even if it is long.

Veterinary models, generally speaking, are lower fidelity and do not offer feedback (e.g. vocalization, pain response, bleeding, bruising). Therefore, feedback must be offered by an observer, so an adequate instructor:student ratio is required for learning to take place in the laboratory. Finally, models – in particular low-fidelity models – are not real, and they require users to suspend their disbelief long enough to take learning seriously and practice their skills (Salas et al., 2005).

The evidence to support the effectiveness of training on models continues to grow at a rapid pace. A meta-analytic review in medical education demonstrated that simulation-based training with deliberate practice yielded better educational outcomes than traditional clinical training, including the model of apprenticeship training that has been medical and veterinary education's paradigm since the start of the 1900s (McGaghie et al., 2011).

Within veterinary clinical skills training specifically, models have proven to be valid and effective at teaching the following skills:

- Surgical hemostasis (Smeak et al., 1991; Olsen et al., 1996; Griffon et al., 2000)
- Canine abdominal laparoscopy (Fransson and Ragle, 2010)
- Rabbit intravenous catheterization (Perez-Rivero and Rendón-Franco, 2011)
- Small animal dental cleaning (Lumbis et al., 2012)
- Equine jugular vein injection (Eichel et al., 2013)
- Equine joint injection (Fox et al., 2013)
- Canine endotracheal intubation and female urinary catheterization (Aulmann et al., 2015)
- Equine nerve block (Gunning et al., 2013)
- Canine intravenous injection (Lee et al., 2013)
- Small animal thoracocentesis (Williamson, 2014)
- Canine ophthalmoscopy (Nibblett et al., 2015)
- Feline abdominal palpation (Williamson et al., 2015)
- Equine intramuscular injection and jugular venipuncture (Williamson et al., 2016)
- Canine castration (Hunt et al., 2020a)
- Bovine castration (Anderson et al., 2020)

- Feline medial saphenous venipuncture (Hunt et al., 2020b)
- Canine dental cleaning (Hunt et al., 2020c)

Many more veterinary models have been described in the literature, often supported by student and expert survey data in favor of their use. Commercially available model options are proliferating as well, though few offer data on learning outcomes (Figure 7.4).

Fidelity

When working with models, the term *fidelity*, or realism, inevitably arises. *Low-fidelity* models are the most common type of models encountered in veterinary medical training. These models, sometimes called task trainers, typically represent only one part of a patient and allow the practice of one or more skills (e.g. practicing venipuncture on a canine forelimb model). Low-fidelity models have traditionally been constructed of materials such as foam, fabric, or wood, although some models may be made of more realistic materials such as silicone. Low-fidelity models are typically utilized for student practice prior to proceeding to live animals and are not generally intended to be a replacement for live animal experience.

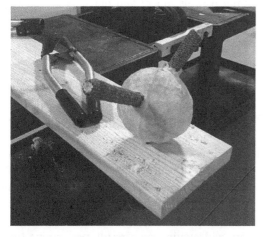

Figure 7.4 The epitome of low fidelity, this frozen cabbage with two corn cobs stands ready to teach students how to use dehorning instruments.

High-fidelity models typically consist of the entire body of a patient or are a realistic representation of a body part or of a specific procedure and are usually constructed of silicone so that they feel realistic as well. These models have sufficient complexity to allow entire procedures or scenarios to be simulated. High-fidelity patient simulators respond to treatment in real time, providing feedback to the student. A few high-fidelity veterinary models have been created (Fletcher et al., 2011; Knight et al., 2014; Yong et al., 2019), while other educators have reported success using high-fidelity human patient simulators in veterinary training scenarios (Modell et al., 2002).

However, fidelity probably exists more as a continuum rather than as two distinct groups – "low" and "high" (Maran and Glavin, 2003). Some authors have recognized this and added the term *medium fidelity* (Gardiner and Oliver, 2014; Zuber et al., 2014;), while others have recommended discarding the term "fidelity" altogether and adopting the terms "physical resemblance" and "functional task alignment" instead (Hamstra et al., 2014). Hamstra (2014) points out that there are multiple facets of fidelity, including whether or not a model looks realistic (*physical resemblance*) and whether or not the model allows for all of the steps of the procedure to be practiced (*functional task alignment*). Models that provide good functional task alignment typically result in good learning outcomes, regardless of their physical resemblance to the live animal (Norman et al., 2012).

When selecting a model to teach skills, educators must take into consideration a variety of factors: features, cost, durability, maintenance and storage requirements, and student and faculty acceptance of the model, among others. Several studies that evaluated veterinary models found that students and educators are more accepting of higher fidelity models (Read et al., 2016; Hunt et al., 2020c). Educational theory suggests that a beginner learner can be trained on a low-fidelity model, but as the learner becomes more advanced, the model should grow in fidelity (Alessi, 1988; American Association of Medical

Colleges, 2007; Brydges et al., 2010). Multiple studies in both human surgery and veterinary surgery have shown that students learn and retain skills just as well when trained on low-fidelity models (Matsumoto et al., 2002; Grober et al., 2004; Read et al., 2016; Williamson et al., 2019). Learning on more simple models may be beneficial because research on the development of motor skills suggests that simulating part of a task may be more beneficial to learning than simulating the entire procedure, as skills are learned as components anyway (Lindahl, 1945; Gagne, 1954; Romiszowski, 1999). Ultimately, the degree of fidelity should be carefully considered based on the level of the student, the educational objectives of the laboratory, and the desired learning outcomes.

Combinations That Work

In veterinary medicine, high-fidelity simulators are scarce and expensive, so the suggestions below leverage lower-fidelity models. These options also fit with the confined budgets faced by many clinical skills programs. If budgets and options allow, higher-fidelity models may also be suitable, keeping in mind that clinical skills programs are often expected to produce measurable outcomes that are commensurate with their cost (Bradley and Bligh, 2005).

Live Animal + Low-Fidelity Model (Simultaneous)

Although live animals are excellent for teaching noninvasive skills, they resent practice of invasive skills or procedures that require aversive tasks to be performed (e.g. indirect ophthalmoscopy, which requires a bright light to be directed into their eyes). In these cases, live animals can be used for the majority of the non-aversive skills practice, such as performing most of a physical examination, where a model would lack an adequate degree of realism. Students can be directed to perform the aversive portions of the examination, such as otoscopy and ophthalmoscopy, on models that have been designed specifically for this purpose.

Low-Fidelity Models, Then Live Animals (Consecutive)

After students have gone through adequate practice on the models to learn the psychomotor skills, instructors then allow them to practice the same procedures on live animals under supervision. Sometimes a gatekeeper assessment will take place between the model and live animal experience to ensure each student's competence and readiness to proceed to live animal work. For example, students may be taught how to perform venipuncture on canine cephalic and jugular vein models prior to performing these procedures on live dogs.

Low-Fidelity Model + High Psychological Fidelity Environment

When a simulation has high psychological fidelity by requiring a similar progression of thought processes necessary on the job, learning has been shown to take place even if the physical realism of the model is low (Bowers and Jentsch, 2001). An example of utilizing this principle would be to take a low-fidelity surgical skills model and put it in a realistic surgical environment where students have to practice a number of perioperative skills using the model. For example, students could be directed to don a cap and mask, perform sterile hand preparation, gown, glove, and enter the surgical theater. Next, students could be directed to drape the model, set up their sterile field, and then perform the surgical procedure on the model using sterile technique. Even though the model itself is a low-fidelity task trainer, the overall learning opportunity has high psychological fidelity because the student must carry out many of the steps that live surgery will require. As a result, performing the surgery "feels real" and significant learning can take place.

Low-Fidelity Model + Simulated Client

Referred to as "patient-focused simulation," this combination allows students to practice interacting with a simulated client in a safe environment while receiving feedback from both a client and clinician on communication skills and clinical skills in the same encounter (Kneebone and Baillie, 2008). This combination creates a richer, more authentic clinical experience for the learner.

Low-Fidelity Model + Cadaver

Low-fidelity models sometimes have limitations regarding anatomy. For example, they may not contain all of the relevant landmarks or structures. If so, presenting them along with an anatomic specimen can be helpful in allowing students to compare the model to the structures present in the real animal.

Ultimately, there is no single combination that heralds clinical skills training success. By incorporating more than one of these teaching modalities, educators can help students benefit from the strengths associated with each. The educational theory of constructivism states that knowledge is not handed intact directly from teacher to student. Instead the student must build their own knowledge and meaning through their learning experiences. Using different teaching tools helps students to build meaning, as it allows students to look at the same topic through a number of different lenses. The variation in teaching methods also helps to keep learning in the clinical skills laboratory from growing predictable and boring.

Regardless of what method is used to teach, an appropriate learning environment is required for skill development. The learning environment impacts cognitive load (Choi et al., 2014) and influences student–instructor and student–peer relationships (Rands and Gansemer-Topf, 2017). When designing clinical skills laboratories, attention should be paid to table arrangements that allow for ease of movement and communication, seating availability, temperature control, noise control, visibility of screens and instructors, and adequate lighting.

Hints for Learning Clinical Skills

Educational theory can be applied to the clinical skills laboratory in order to gain insight into how a student can best learn clinical skills. Fitts and Posner (1967) described how motor skills are learned in three steps: *cognition*, *integration*, and *automation*. The first step, *cognition*, is the understanding of how to do something, which is typically accomplished by watching a demonstration of the task, whether recorded or live, or reading a description of the procedure. Notes may be helpful if the task is in depth, or a sketch if suture patterns or surgical approaches are involved. *Integration* is the stage in which most students spend the bulk of their time, practicing the skills but having to continuously concentrate on the task and how to improve their performance. The key here is to observe their own performance and ask others for feedback on it. The third step, *automation*, occurs later when minimal concentration and effort are needed. Usually, this is only achieved once significant practice has been undertaken.

Bandura (1986) described social cognitive theory, which states that students remain motivated to learn from one another by observing and imitating modeled behaviors. In other words, students who look to their instructors and fellow students in order to find performances that are a stronger than their own will often find motivation to keep working to improve their skills. This is in contrast to the student who becomes satisfied and complacent with their own skill set and stops growing. Caution should also be issued against finding someone whose skill set is immensely superior and despairing at the inequality, as that is also unhelpful. Skills are grown sequentially and finding someone whose skills are modestly better to look to is often a better choice.

Knowles (1975) explained the concept of self-directed learning as the process learners take in setting their own learning goals, identifying their own resources, and evaluating their learning gains. Veterinary students are adult learners, which means that they are largely driven by *intrinsic*, rather than *extrinsic*, motivation. In other words, they learn because they recognize a need for learning. This is important because, as advances continue to be made in veterinary medicine, they will be able to continue to learn new things throughout their careers. Therefore, being capable of self-directed learning is critical to their professional success both in learning clinical skills initially and in remaining a competent practitioner over the course of their career. Setting learning goals that are meaningful to them and identifying and utilizing available resources are very important in enhancing clinical skills learning.

Finally, deliberate practice as described by Ericsson (2004) is extremely relevant to achieving competence in clinical skills. Psychomotor skills such as administering medicine, drawing blood, performing a physical examination, or performing surgery are learned through repetitive practice with rigorous skills assessment and specific feedback. In the clinical skills laboratory, this means that students should be prepared to put in the hours of practice that are required to become competent and not to expect short cuts to competence. Practice time is best spaced over a period of several weeks or months, not massed into a few intensive days (Moulton et al., 2006). Students should seek out feedback as frequently as possible so that they can continue to grow their skills efficiently and accurately. In fact, provision of feedback was the strongest predictor of success in a meta-analysis of simulation-based training, more than the features of the model or any other single factor (Issenberg et al., 2005).

Conclusions

The transition of veterinary training from a purely apprenticeship model to a clinical skills program *plus* clinical training phase has much to offer the student. Modern clinical skills curricula frequently make use of a combination of live animals, cadaver tissue, and models of varying fidelity in order to meet the educational needs of students, both in teaching and in assessment. Even experienced educators may be challenged to structure a well-designed program that thoughtfully weaves together the different educational methods in a way that reinforces each other with planned repetition to support student skill development and encourage retention, along with assessments to gauge student progress, and remediation opportunities for students who fail to meet benchmark criteria.

A Clinical Skills Training Example

The authors have chosen to share an example of how clinical skills curriculum is structured at their institution, and how one specific skill – handling of companion animals – is taught in that curriculum. This example is being used to illustrate how multiple methods of instruction (models and live animals) can be brought together to teach a single skill set, how assessment can be built into multiple levels of a program, how the requirements of deliberate practice (repetition and feedback) can be achieved, and how complexity can be built over time.

General Course Information

Lincoln Memorial University College of Veterinary Medicine (LMU CVM) has designed a comprehensive clinical skills curriculum as a way for students to progressively gain hands-on experience. The clinical skills curriculum consists of six semesters of mandatory, letter-graded courses that students must pass to progress through the veterinary curriculum.

During each Clinical Skills lab, students are given time to practice skills under supervision and are given targeted advice according to the principles of effective feedback (Nicol and Macfarlane-Dick, 2006; Cornell, 2017). At the end of the session, students are individually assessed on their ability to perform a selected skill. Each student is given feedback about what was performed well, informed where there was room for additional improvement, and assigned a Global Rating Score using a six-point scale (1 = very poor, 2 = poor, 3 = borderline unsatisfactory, 4 = borderline satisfactory, 5 = good, 6 = excellent). Scores of 4–6 are considered passing scores, while scores of 1–3 are considered not to have met minimum expectations. Points received from these assessments are combined with online or in-laboratory knowledge-based quizzes and objective structured clinical examinations (OSCEs) each semester to generate a student's course grade. Students are strongly encouraged to practice their skills outside of scheduled laboratory sessions, and they are provided with a well-stocked practice laboratory space and models to take home to facilitate practice.

Delivery of the Gentle Animal Handling Curriculum

Gentle animal handling techniques decrease the fear, anxiety, and stress felt by companion animals during veterinary visits. The authors teach these techniques to veterinary students using models and live animals in a series of laboratories, each reviewing and building on content previously presented. Students' deliberate practice is meant to build, refine, and reinforce gentle animal handling skills from the start of their veterinary education in order to prepare them to gently handle animals during their clinical year and beyond.

Clinical Skills laboratory (CSL) sessions are taught by veterinarians and, when appropriate for the skill, veterinary technicians (nurses). Prior to teaching in the CSL, instructors attend a presentation emphasizing the delivery of quality feedback and reach consensus on how to teach gentle animal handling skills through a series of meetings or workshops that allow discussion and practice of skills (Johnson and Williamson, 2018). Students are required to review pre-laboratory materials such as videos or reading before attending the CSL. Students are required to complete the online Fear Free certification course (https://fearfreepets.com/fear-free-certification-overview/) prior to handling companion animals in the first semester of their veterinary program. Students subsequently practice gentle animal handling through a series of progressive CSL sessions in semesters 1–6. These sessions use a combination of models and live dogs and cats (Table 7.1).

Sessions contain animal handling practice exclusively so that students only focus on handling tasks. Some of these tasks can be practiced on models, such as tasks including how to pick up dogs while providing proper support to the hind end, how to apply and adjust a muzzle, how to utilize a rabies pole, and how to restrain for venipuncture without performing it. Other tasks such as behavioral assessment can only be practiced on live dogs. As students progress through the curriculum, they are expected to utilize these gentle handling skills while performing other tasks on live animals, such as performing a physical examination, drawing blood, explaining physical examination findings to a client, or working up a surgical patient. In this way, complexity is added to the student's task and the student grows in his/her ability to function at the level expected of a new veterinarian, which is to be able to simultaneously handle an animal while performing a task on the animal.

In laboratory sessions that include both models and live animals, students start by practicing their skills on the models in order to receive feedback and refine their technique. Once they have reached proficiency and feel comfortable with the tasks they are to perform, they are assigned live animals to work with. In the earlier semesters, when students are still learning and practicing their skills, their live animal work is exclusively on dogs, which are generally easier to handle than cats. As students grow in skill, eventually handling sessions with live, cooperative pet cats are added. Finally, in sixth semester, students begin to handle shelter dogs and cats, whose

Table 7.1 LMU CVM clinical skills laboratories with gentle animal handling content. All laboratories are approved by the Institutional Animal Care and Use Committee (IACUC) and are performed under direct faculty supervision.

Semester	Lab title	Species	Live animal use	Model use
1	Canine Handling	Canine	X	X
	Feline Handling	Feline		X
	Introduction to Canine Physical Examination	Canine	X	X
2	Canine Physical Examination II	Canine	X	
	Canine Venipuncture	Canine	X	X
3	Canine Physical Examination III – Focus on Ophthalmology & Oral Cavity	Canine	X	X
	Basic Clicker Training	Canine	X	
4	Communication Skills & the Physical Examination	Canine	X	
5	Canine Fear Free Handling	Canine	X	
	Surgery Work Up – Examination & Diagnostics	Canine	X	
6	Feline Fear Free Handling	Feline	X	
	Canine Physical Examination IV – Focus on Ophthalmology with Fundic Exam & Otoscopy	Canine	X	X
	Surgery Patient Work Up – Examination & Diagnostics	Canine & Feline	X	

temperaments may add an additional degree of challenge.

The progression of these laboratories is designed to teach students to perform gentle animal handling and allow them the opportunity to practice these skills repetitively with an increasing level of difficulty and complexity. As the level of difficulty increases, students recognize progression in their journey toward becoming veterinarians, but do not become overwhelmed by being expected to be instantly competent at the most difficult tasks, such as handling shelter cats adeptly, on their first day of class.

Discussion of the Gentle Animal Handling Curriculum

The progressive series of clinical skills laboratories described represent a spiral curriculum, where skills are taught and expanded upon over time to reinforce previous content and integrate new information and skills (Harden and Stamper, 1999). Most veterinary students have an interest in pursuing companion animal medicine as a career (*AVMA Market Research Statistics*, 2018), so they are intrinsically motivated to learn these techniques. Students are also motivated by the OSCE they must pass once a semester in order to progress through the curriculum.

Delivery of these clinical skills sessions has not been without its challenges. First, there are diverse handling methods taught and used within the veterinary profession, and this was true among the veterinarians and technicians (nurses) employed by LMU. However, we understood while designing the clinical skills program that reaching consensus among the educators and clinicians would be critical. If we taught students gentle techniques in their handling labs during their first two semesters, only for them to observe clinicians performing conflicting handling methods during surgery patient work-up in semesters five and six, students would soon learn that animals are treated differently whenever the situation requires it. We assembled the relevant faculty and underwent a series of discussions to build consensus, eventually reaching the conclusion to teach and practice gentle handling methods in our facility. We began hosting workshops for faculty to practice gentle handling techniques on dogs and cats, to ask questions, and to discuss available training. A number of the faculty chose to become Fear Free-certified.

Another challenge we face is that many students begin veterinary school thinking that they already know how to handle dogs and cats correctly. Helping students to realize that they are not yet fully skilled at reading canine and feline body language and interpreting how they should proceed for the best possible outcome can be a challenge. Students with more handling experience can be particularly difficult to convince to adopt a new and different method. Faculty presenting a united message that these are the handling techniques that will be used in this facility, and included in our assessments, is critical to convincing students to learn new methods.

A further challenge has been having our students learn these techniques using shelter animals that exhibit a range of fear, anxiety, and stress (FAS) levels, resulting in the students' experiences sometimes being inconsistent. However, handling a variety of patients is similar to what students may encounter in a veterinary practice. Some of the dogs we have worked with in the clinical skills laboratory are not fearful, anxious, or stressed and only need treats as a reward for calm behavior, especially younger dogs. Some students have struggled to recognize this, and dogs may be given treats inappropriately and inadvertently taught to chase hands. Students are encouraged to learn to increase treat value based on FAS levels and patient reaction to procedures rather than merely giving many treats at once.

LMU CVM has been both limited and bolstered by having a small but growing faculty that is highly involved in clinical skills laboratories. Having a relatively new program means there has been less opportunity to gather data and make changes to the existing curriculum, but it also means there is more ability to make adjustments. Every program that institutes clinical skills training has its own unique strengths and potential pitfalls. Predicting these and addressing them, while remaining open to truthful re-evaluation and adjustment, will only support a program's success.

References

Alessi, S. M. 1988. Fidelity in the design of instructional simulations. *JCBI*, 15, 40–47.

American Association of Medical Colleges. 2007. Effective Use of Educational Technology in Medical Education. https://store.aamc.org/effective-use-of-educational-technology-in-medical-education-pdf.html Accessed February 14, 2021.

Anderson, S. L., Miller, L., Gibbons, P., et al. 2020. Development and validation of a bovine castration model and rubric. *J Vet Med Educ*, Feb 13, e20180016.

Aulmann, M., März, M., Burgener, I. A., et al. 2015. Development and evaluation of two canine low-fidelity simulation models. *J Vet Med Educ*, 42, 151–160.

AVMA Market Research Statistics. 2018. *Market Research Statistics*. Schaumburg, IL: American Association of Veterinary Medicine.

Bandura, A. 1986. *Social Foundations of Thought and Action: A Social Cognitive Theory*. Englewood Cliffs, NJ: Prentice Hall.

Bowers, C. A., Jentsch, F. 2001. Use of commercial, off-the-shelf, simulations for team research. In: *Advances in Human Performance and Cognitive Engineering Research*, Vol. 1. Salas, E. (ed.) Bingley, UK: Emerald Publishing, pp. 293–317.

Bradley, P., Bligh, J. 2005. Clinical skills centres: Where are we going? *Med Educ*, 39, 649–650.

Brydges, R., Carnahan, H., Rose, D., et al. 2010. Coordinating progressive levels of simulation fidelity to maximize educational benefit. *Acad Med*, 85, 806–812.

Choi, H. H., van Merriënboer, J. J. G., Paas, F. 2014. Effects of the physical environment on cognitive load and learning: Towards a new model of cognitive load. *Educ Psychol Rev*, 26, 225–244.

Cornell, K. 2017. Feedback in veterinary medical education. In: *Veterinary Medical Education: A Practical Guide*. Hodgson, J. L., Pelzer, J. M. (eds.) Hoboken, NJ: Wiley and Sons, Inc., pp. 273–285.

Eichel, J.-C., Korb, W., Schlenker, A., et al. 2013. Evaluation of a training model to teach veterinary students a technique for injecting the jugular vein in horses. *J Vet Med Educ*, 40, 288–295.

Ericsson, K. A. 2004. Deliberate practice and the acquisition and maintenance of expert performance in medicine and related domains. *Acad Med*, 79, S70–S81.

Fitts, P., Posner, M. 1967. *Human Performance*. Belmont, CA: Brooks/Cole.

Fletcher, D. J., Militello, R., Schoeffler, G. L., et al. 2011. Development and evaluation of a high-fidelity canine patient simulator for veterinary clinical training. *J Vet Med Educ*, 39, 7–12.

Fox, V., Sinclair, C., Bolt, D. M., et al. 2013. Design and validation of a simulator for equine joint injections. *J Vet Med Educ*, 40, 152–157.

Fransson, B. A., Ragle, C. A. 2010. Assessment of laparoscopic skills before and after simulation training with a canine abdominal model. *J Am Vet Med Assoc*, 236, 1079–1084.

Gagne, R. M. 1954. Training devices and simulators: some research issues. *Am Psychol*, 9, 95–107.

Gardiner, A., Oliver, F. 2014. Low- and medium-fidelity models for core skills in dentistry. VetEd 2014, 2014, Bristol, UK, p. 11.

Griffon, D. J., Cronin, P., Kirby, B., et al. 2000. Evaluation of a hemostasis model for teaching ovariohysterectomy in veterinary surgery', *Vet Surg*, 29, 309–316.

Grober, E. D., Hamstra, S. J., Wanzel, K. R., et al. 2004. The educational impact of bench model fidelity on the acquisition of technical skill: The use of clinically relevant outcome measures. *Ann Surg*, 24, 374–381.

Gunning, P., Smith, A., Fox, V., et al. 2013. Development and validation of an equine nerve block simulator to supplement practical skills training in undergraduate veterinary students. *Vet Rec*, 172, 450.

Halsted, W. S. 1904. The training of the surgeon. *JAMA*, 18, 1553–1554.

Hamstra, S. J., Brydges, R., Hatala, R., et al. 2014. Reconsidering fidelity in simulation-based training. *Acad Med*, 89, 387–392.

Harden, R., Stamper, N. 1999. What is a spiral curriculum? *Med Teach*, 21, 141–143.

Hunt, J. A., Heydejburg, M., Kelly, C. K., et al. 2020a. Development and validation of a canine castration model and rubric', *J Vet Med Educ*, 47, 78–90.

Hunt, J. A., Hughes, C., Asciutto, M., et al. 2020b. Development and validation of a feline medial saphenous venipuncture model and rubric. *J Vet Med Educ*, 47, 333–341.

Hunt, J. A., Schmidt, P., Perkins, J., et al. 2020c. Comparison of three canine models for teaching veterinary dental cleaning. *J Vet Med Educ*, Advance Online, e20200001. doi: https://doi.org/10.3138/jvme-2020-0001.

Issenberg, S. B., McGaghie, W. C., Petrusa, E. R., et al. 2005. Features and uses of high-fidelity medical simulations that lead to effective learning: A BEME systematic review. *Med Teach*, 27, 10–28.

Johnson, J., Williamson, J. 2018. Faculty development with integration of low stress pet handling techniques into a veterinary school curriculum, *MedEdPublish*, 7, 52.

Kneebone, R., Baillie, S. 2008. Contextualized simulation and procedural skills: A view from medical education. *J Vet Med Educ*, 35, 595–598.

Knight, A., Bauman, E., Pederson, D, et al. 2014. The birth of "SimDonkey": the development of a high fidelity donkey patient simulator. (Poster) World Congress on Alternatives and Animal Use in the Life Sciences, Prague.

Knowles, M. S. 1975. *Self-Directed Learning: A Guide for Learners and Teachers*. New York, NY: Association Press.

Langebæk, R., Eika, B., Jensen, A. L., et al. 2012a. Anxiety in veterinary surgical students: A quantitative study. *J Vet Med Educ*, 39, 331–340.

Langebæk, R, Eika, B., Tangaard, L., et al. 2012b. Emotions in veterinary surgical students: A qualitative study. *J Vet Med Educ*, 39, 312–321.

Lee, S., Lee, J., Park, N., et al. 2013. Augmented reality intravenous injection simulator based 3D medical imaging for veterinary medicine. *Vet J*, 196, 197–202.

Lindahl, L. G. 1945. Movement analysis as an industrial training method. *J Appl Psychol*, 29, 420–436.

Lumbis, R. H., Gregory, S. P., Baillie, S. 2012. Evaluation of a dental model for training veterinary students. *J Vet Med Educ*, 39, 128–135.

Maran, N. J., Glavin, R. J. 2003. Low- to high-fidelity simulation - a continuum of medical education? *Med Educ*, 37, 22–28.

Matsumoto, E. D., Hamstra, S. J., Radomski, S. B., et al. 2002. The effect of bench model fidelity on endourological skills: A randomized controlled study. *J Urol*, 167, 1243–1247.

McGaghie, W. C., Issenberg, S. B., Cohen, E. R., et al. 2011. Does simulation-based medical education with deliberate practice yield better results than traditional clinical education? A meta-analytic comparative review of the evidence. *Acad Med*, 86, 706–711.

Modell, J. H., Cantwell, S., Hardcastle, J., et al. 2002. Using the human patient simulator to educate students of veterinary medicine. *J Vet Med Educ*, 29, 111–116.

Moulton, C.-A. E., Dubrowski, A., Macrae, H., et al. 2006. Teaching surgical skills: What kind of practice makes perfect? *Ann Surg*, 244, 400–409.

Nibblett, B. M. D., Pereira, M. M., Williamson, J. A., et al. 2015. Validation of a model for teaching canine fundoscopy. *J Vet Med Educ*, 42, 133–139.

Nicol, D. J., Macfarlane-Dick, D. 2006. Formative assessment and self-regulated learning: A model and seven principles of good feedback practice. *Stud High Educ*, 31, 199–218.

Norman, G., Dore, K., Grierson, L. 2012. The minimal relationship between simulation fidelity and transfer of learning. *Med Educ*, 46, 636–647.

Olsen, D., Bauer, M. S., Seim, H. B., et al. 1996. Evaluation of a hemostasis model for teaching basic surgical skills. *Vet Surg*, 25, 49–58.

Perez-Rivero, J. J., Rendón-Franco, E. 2011. Validation of the educational potential of a simulator to develop abilities and skills for the creation and maintenance of an intravenous cannula. *Altern Lab Anim*, 39, 257–260.

Rands, M., Gansemer-Topf, A. 2017. "The room itself is active": How classroom design impacts student engagement. *J Learn. Spaces*, 6, 26–33.

Read, E. K., Vallevand, A., Farrell, R. M. 2016. Evaluation of veterinary student surgical skills preparation for ovariohysterectomy using simulators: A pilot study. *J Vet Med Educ*, 43, 190–213.

Romiszowski, A. 1999. The development of physical skills: Instruction in the psychomotor domain. In: *Instructional-Design Theories and Models: A New Paradigm of Instructional Theory*. Reigeluth, C. M. (ed.) Mahwah, NJ: Lawrence Erlbaum Associates, pp. 460–481.

Salas, E., Wilson, K. A., Burke, C. S., et al. 2005. Using simulation-based training to improve patient safety: What does it take? *Jt Comm J Qual Patient Saf*, 31, 363–371.

Smeak, D. D., Beck, M. L., Shaffer, C. A., et al. 1991. Evaluation of video tape and a simulator for instruction of basic surgical skills. *Vet Surg*, 20, 30–36.

Williamson, J. A. 2014. Construct validation of a small-animal thoracocentesis simulator. *V Vet Med Educ*, 41, 384–389.

Williamson, J. A., Hecker, K., Yvorchuk, K., et al. 2015. Development and validation of a feline abdominal palpation model and scoring rubric. *Vet Rec*, 177, 151.

Williamson, J. A., Dascanio, J. J., Christmann, U., et al. 2016. Development and validation of a model for training equine phlebotomy and intramuscular injection skills. *J Vet Med Educ*, 43, 235–242.

Williamson, J. A., Brisson, B. A., Anderson, S. L., et al. 2019. Comparison of 2 canine celiotomy closure models for training novice veterinary students. *Vet Surg*, 48, 966–974.

Yong, J. A. A., Kim, S. E., Case, J. B. 2019. Survey of clinician and student impressions of a synthetic canine model for gastrointestinal surgery training. *Vet Surg*, 48, 343–351.

Zuber, M., Matthew, S., Hannan, N. et al. 2014. Evaluation of a medium fidelity dog spay simulation model. Poster presented at 5th Veterinary Education Symposium. July 10-11, 2014, University of Bristol. Bristol, UK.

8

How Do I Make Use of Peer Teaching?

Lucy Squire[1] and Marc Dilly[2]

[1] *Bristol Veterinary School, University of Bristol, Bristol, UK*
[2] *Faculty of Veterinary Medicine, Justus Liebig, University Giessen, Giessen, Germany*

Key Messages

- Peer-assisted learning (PAL) is a generic term for strategies that involve the interactive process of learning through other learners who are not "professional" teachers
- PAL can be used to teach various clinical skills, including clinical examinations, suturing, injections, and intravenous catheter placement
- The use of PAL has many benefits for the student tutor, the student tutee, and the institution itself. Student tutors often stand to benefit the most from PAL
- Student tutor knowledge and training are cited as limitations of PAL, alongside difficulties with logistics and timetabling, but these can be managed with tutor training and careful planning

- PAL can be used across different cohorts or between students in the same academic year, and can be optional or compulsory
- PAL is used to provide feedback and multiple chances for learning and to develop student competences. It can provide resources for assessments and preparation for examinations
- Training of student tutors is essential for successful PAL. It can be helpful to provide structure for student tutors involved in PAL, keep group sizes small, and ensure the atmosphere is informal

---

Introduction

Peer teaching and learning formats have been reported since the 1960s and 1970s (Goldschmid and Goldschmid, 1976; Devin-Sheehan et al., 1976). Within the last 30 years, they have been gaining in importance and undergone considerable development in several disciplines including the health professions. This is reflected in an increase and abundance of published literature; in the last six years alone, more than 250 publications on peer teaching have been published on PubMed (ten Cate, 2017).

Veterinary Clinical Skills, First Edition. Edited by Emma K. Read, Matt R. Read, and Sarah Baillie.
© 2022 John Wiley & Sons, Inc. Published 2022 by John Wiley & Sons, Inc.
Companion website: www.wiley.com/go/read/veterinary

Peer teaching can be defined as the development of knowledge and skills through explicit active support of other students, with the deliberate intent to help others with their learning goals (Topping and Ehly, 2001). Recognized as an enriching and effective learning method for students (Tolsgaard et al., 2007; Weyrich et al., 2008; Evans and Cuffe, 2009; Benè and Bergus, 2014), peer teaching is being used widely across the healthcare professions. For example, peer teaching is described in medicine (Soriano et al., 2010; Seenan et al., 2016; Alvarez et al., 2017), as well as in nursing (Morris and Turnbull, 2004; Zentz et al., 2014), in dentistry (Brueckner and MacPherson, 2004), in veterinary medicine (Monahan and Yew, 2002; Baillie et al., 2009; Engelskirchen et al., 2017), physiotherapy (Solomon and Crowe, 2001), in osteopathy (McWhorter and Forester, 2004), psychology (Fantuzzo et al., 1989), and pharmacy (Aburahma and Mohamed, 2017).

What Is Peer Teaching?

The terms *peer teaching* and *peer-assisted learning* (PAL) are often used synonymously (Yu et al., 2011). For the readability of this chapter, the term PAL will be used. *Peer-tutoring* is also used occasionally, but more commonly refers to one-to-one teaching (ten Cate and Durning, 2007a).

PAL is a generic term for strategies that involve the interactive process of learning from other learners who are not "professional" teachers (Topping and Ehly, 2001). In this scenario, the peer teachers are referred to as "tutors" and the learners are referred to as "tutees." Tutors have a deliberate intent to help their tutees, who are mostly of an equal status. Most tutors are from the same cohort or a higher year. They help their tutees learn and expand their own abilities in a "cooperative learning" setting (Topping, 2005). The main features of PAL are tutors assisting tutees to learn (and in so doing, learning themselves); the teaching and learning is structured to ensure benefits for all participants; it is supported and monitored by professional teachers.

Different PAL formats can be described based on three criteria (ten Cate and Durning, 2007a). First, it is possible to differentiate tutors as "same-level" and "near-year or cross-year" in comparison to their tutees. "Same-level" means that there is little or no difference between the level of education of the tutors and the tutees (e.g. Team Based Learning described by Michaelsen and Sweet, 2011). In "near-year or cross-year," the tutor is at least a year ahead of the tutees (ten Cate and Durning, 2007a; Hammond et al., 2010). Second, the size of the study group or the ratio of tutors to tutees can be classified as a criterion. Due to the variety of intended learning outcomes (knowledge, skills, attitudes), there are several suitable ratios. For example, in the context of technical–practical skills, a ratio of one tutor to four tutees is optimal (Dubrowski and MacRae, 2006). The third criterion is the formality of the setting in which the peer teaching takes place. On one hand, the tutors and tutees can meet in a more or less informal private setting (e.g. in the library, in a skills lab, or collaborate via social media). On the other hand, the university may organize and schedule courses for peer teaching with or without supervision by lecturers (ten Cate and Durning, 2007a). All arrangements aim to encourage cooperative learning and foster competences of students.

PAL has been shown to be well received by students and tutors and is an enriching learning method for students (Topping, 2005; Baillie et al., 2009). Moreover, teaching and learning are important professional attributes, which is why medical schools are increasingly seeking to train young doctors as competent teachers (Fincher et al., 2000). PAL can also strengthen the interest in an academic career (ten Cate and Durning, 2007a) and provide opportunities for the development of several competences (e.g. communication, self-reflection, providing feedback, etc.).

The next section will discuss the benefits and limitations of PAL, before describing how to implement PAL. Due to the progressive inclusion of PAL in curricula (Alvarez et al., 2017), validating and measuring its effectiveness is important. In a review by Yu et al. (2011), 10 out of 12 studies showed a similar learning outcome between PAL and traditional formats.

What Are the Benefits and Limitations of Peer-assisted Learning?

Benefits of PAL

There are many recognized benefits of PAL, for the tutor, the tutee and the institution (Table 8.1).

Benefits for Student Tutors

One of the benefits of PAL is that students learn how to teach. This is an important skill to develop. Once qualified, veterinarians and veterinary nurses will be teaching and delivering information on a daily basis to a varied audience that might include veterinary colleagues, staff members, animals owners and other stakeholders. This will occur informally, for example when explaining concepts and treatment plans, and more explicitly, for example teaching an owner how to deliver a subcutaneous injection to a diabetic cat. There is also workplace-based teaching of veterinary and nursing students, in both primary care practices and a referral setting. While teaching is not a Day One competency in the veterinary profession (RCVS, 2020), our medical counterparts value it highly enough to have it stated as a requirement of all newly qualified doctors (GMC, 2018).

There are many examples of PAL initiatives in which students feel they have developed their teaching skills as a result of being a tutor (Baillie et al., 2009; Burgess et al., 2012; Bates et al., 2016). While it is difficult to directly measure whether teaching skills have developed as a result of participating in a PAL program, quotes from student tutors include "I have learnt how to explain things in a way people will understand," suggesting that students are, in fact, developing relevant skills (Bates et al., 2016).

It seems relatively obvious that students would develop their teaching skills as a result of participating in a PAL program. In addition, many programs provide some sort of training for their tutors, enabling them to deliver the sessions effectively and ensuring they get the most out of the program (Baillie et al., 2009; Burgess et al., 2012; Bates et al., 2016). Additionally, the tutors get the opportunity to practice these teaching skills during PAL sessions, when the emphasis is on the process of teaching, rather than solely on knowledge.

Related to the development of teaching skills, tutors also develop their communication skills. While there is much overlap between teaching skills and communication skills, when asked about the benefits of participating in PAL programs, students specify improvements in communication (Krych et al., 2005; Bell et al., 2017), teaching (Burgess et al., 2012), or both (Dandavino et al., 2007; Baillie et al., 2009; Bates et al., 2016), indicating that students do see these skills as different. Communication skills are known to be important in the veterinary profession, not only for communicating with clients but also with colleagues. Any opportunity to develop these skills can be seen as an advantage. As for teaching skills, it is difficult to directly

Table 8.1 Benefits of PAL.

Tutor	Tutee	Institution
Learn how to teach	Safe environment	Less staff time required
Improve communication skills	Relatable tutor	Exposure of young professionals to teaching and learning strategies
Deepen own understanding	Smaller groups than core teaching	
Increase confidence	Meet students from other years	Smaller group sizes – supplement teaching staff
Form professional identity		
Develop learning skills		
Develop leadership skills		

assess whether students are actually improving their communication skills, or if this is merely a perception on their part, but it is a potential benefit.

Another benefit for tutors involved in PAL is the deepening of knowledge in the subject area. For example, Peets et al. (2009) found students performed better on multiple choice questions on subjects which they had taught, compared to questions in the same exam on which they had been tutees. It seems logical that students would develop their own knowledge as a result of teaching – one must understand a topic well in order to be able to teach it. Tutors in a veterinary PAL program indicated that participating in a PAL activity had allowed them to identify their own strengths and weaknesses, an important factor in filling gaps in knowledge (Bell et al., 2017). Peets et al. (2009), also reported that students spent much longer preparing for sessions on which they would teach, compared to sessions on which they would be passive learners. This is likely to also contribute to an increase in knowledge and test performance.

An increase in self-confidence has been mentioned in some PAL programs. For example, tutors reported an increase in confidence as a result of teaching others (Baillie et al., 2009; Bates et al., 2016; Bell et al., 2017) and a decrease in anxiety and self-doubt (Weyrich et al., 2008). This increase in confidence is reflected in a statement from a tutor in a PAL program, who commented that "I've realised you know more than you think you do" (Bates et al., 2016).

When PAL is included in the formal curriculum, it may also help with professional identity formation. Students will each have a view of what it means to be a veterinarian and, while this will frequently involve teaching, not all students will see "teacher" as part of their professional identity. In fact, Amorosa et al. (2011) describe how students do not realize that teaching is an important part of being a clinician until they have been involved in teaching themselves. In teaching students how to teach, we are making explicit the importance of this skill and indicating to students it is something to be valued and one of the many skills needed to be a well-rounded clinician. Following PAL training, a senior medical student stated "I'd see teaching as part of my job after the course we've just done" (Burgess et al., 2012). Teaching students about teaching helps them to recognize it as part of their identity which, in turn, may help them to value the skill more when they have to teach in practice (Dandavino et al., 2007).

Other benefits for PAL tutors include developing their own learning skills. Senior medical students on a PAL training course reported a significant improvement in their perceived understanding of educational principles, with one student stating "*I think [the course] taught us how to be a better learner*" (Burgess et al., 2012). Some tutors have also mentioned an increase in leadership skills (ten Cate and Durning, 2007b; Weyrich et al., 2008).

Benefits for Student Tutees

Tutees also stand to benefit from being taught by student tutors rather than academic staff. Tutees in PAL programs frequently refer to there being a less intimidating and safer learning atmosphere compared to sessions taught by staff, with students on a veterinary PAL program referring to the "approachability" of the student tutors (Bulte et al., 2007; Weyrich et al., 2008; Baillie et al., 2009; Bates et al., 2016; Bell et al., 2017). As the teaching style is less authoritarian, students report that the learning atmosphere is more pleasant and less stressful than traditional lecture-based courses (ten Cate and Durning, 2007b; Baillie et al., 2009). This can lead to an increase in self-confidence in the learners and can foster competence development (Agius et al., 2018). Additionally, an informal atmosphere may stimulate more interaction between the tutee and tutor and tutees feel able to "ask silly questions," thus potentially deepening their understanding in a way that may not happen if being taught by staff (Bulte et al., 2007; Bates et al., 2016).

One of the most positive effects of PAL is the social and cognitive congruence that exists between tutors and tutees (Schmidt and Moust, 1995; Lockspeiser et al., 2008; Benè and Bergus, 2014). Socially and cognitively minded individuals are usually better able to understand the situation of the learners and understand their problems. Student tutees find that student tutors are more relatable than academic staff (Baillie et al., 2009; Bates et al., 2016; Bell et al., 2017). This means that tutors may be better able to explain things in a way that is accessible for the tutees (Bell et al., 2017). This is because tutors may have a better understanding of the aspects that are likely to be difficult and are better at "highlighting key points" (Bulte et al., 2007; Baillie et al., 2009; Bates et al., 2016). As a veterinary student tutee in a PAL program stated, "they can remember how it felt this time last year" (Bates et al., 2016).

When compared to group learning in the curriculum taught by academics, some PAL programs have the added benefit of having smaller tutee group sizes (Weyrich et al., 2008; Baillie et al., 2009; Bates et al., 2016). This increased ratio of tutor to tutee can allow for more effective feedback on technique and maximize learning by tutees (Weyrich et al., 2008).

Finally, some programs mention that PAL programs enable students at different stages of the curriculum to meet each other, which can have additional benefits. Some veterinary tutees on PAL programs simply appreciated the opportunity to meet students from higher years and the chance to discuss various aspects of the program with them, while others mention more specifically being able to ask student tutors about study skills in a way that they would not ask academic staff (Bulte et al., 2007; Bell et al., 2017).

Benefits for the Institution

Many of the benefits applicable to tutors and tutees will also apply to the institution; institutions gain from students learning in smaller group sizes, developing increased communication and teaching skills, and having better awareness of different teaching and learning strategies.

Institutions may also benefit from using a PAL program since PAL can be a way to supplement teaching and learning without the need for additional staff - saving time and resources (Ross and Cameron, 2007; Baillie et al., 2009; Strand et al., 2013). As student numbers increase in many veterinary schools, PAL may provide a way to keep group sizes small without the need for equivalent increases in staff (Topping, 1996). In a medical PAL program involving skills lab training, 85% of tutees responded that training from student tutors alone was adequate (Weyrich et al., 2008). However, it is worth considering that tutor training is recommended, and while there is the potential for less staff input in the teaching, the provision of training, and organization of the PAL program can be time-intensive. Ross and Cameron (2007) also discuss the ethical considerations around using a PAL program. While a reduction in staff resources may be a reasonable benefit, this should not be the main reason PAL is incorporated into a program.

Limitations of PAL

As we have discussed above, PAL has many benefits, but it is important to also be aware of its main limitations, namely, the level of knowledge of the tutor, the teaching experience of the tutor, and timing and logistics. Many of these limitations can be managed with appropriate training of tutors and planning in general (see "How to implement PAL" below for more information).

A frequently referenced limitation of PAL is the level of knowledge of the peer tutor. This is cited by both tutees and tutors, as well as by staff within the institution, who believe it is inappropriate for students to teach other students (Bulte et al., 2007; Ross and Cameron, 2007; Weyrich et al., 2008; Baillie et al., 2009; Bates et al., 2016). In addition to having a lower level of knowledge than academic staff, student tutors have less clinical experience and so are less able to use examples to help illustrate challenging points (Bulte et al., 2007). This can be a particular problem with tutors at the same academic level as the tutees, as there may be minimal difference in knowledge (Baillie et al., 2009). However, it should be considered that this lesser knowledge also contributes to some of the benefits of PAL, such as tutors being less intimidating and better able to empathize with difficult concepts, as described above.

The limited teaching experience of the peer tutors is also often mentioned as a potential disadvantage to PAL. While it is recommended that peer tutors undergo training before starting to teach other students, students still lack the level of experience of staff (Ross and Cameron, 2007). This can result in a variety of difficulties. For example, student tutors may immediately answer a more difficult question, rather than waiting and then leading tutees to work out the answer for themselves, an approach typical of a more experienced teacher (Bulte et al., 2007). Due to their lack of clinical experience and/or their similar age and lack of seniority, tutors may also find it difficult to motivate students (Bulte et al., 2007). This may result in difficulty creating order and respect in a teaching session (Bulte et al., 2007; Weyrich et al., 2008). Ross and Cameron (2007) discuss how inexperience in teaching may lead tutors to overload tutees with information. As for tutor knowledge, some of these limitations are also linked to the benefits of PAL, as the lack of seniority helps to contribute to the informal learning environment, so a balance needs to be met.

Time and logistics can also be limitations for creating a PAL program or unit within a curriculum. While decreasing staff time and input is a potential benefit of PAL, the initial set-up can still be time-consuming and require a lot of staff input (e.g. planning the session, training tutors, creating resources, and answering tutor queries) (Ross and Cameron, 2007).

How to Use and Implement Peer Teaching

Teaching Methods for PAL

Various teaching methods can be used in the context of peer teaching. Common to all types, the learning outcomes are greatest when previously defined learning goals are clearly communicated

to both the tutors and tutees (Issenberg et al., 2005). For the mastery of psychomotor skills in medicine, it is essential that students pass through and complete three consecutive learning stages: the action to be learned should be closely observed being performed by the instructor, then it is performed under supervision multiple times before eventually being performed by the learner independently and routinely (Schnabel et al., 2011). This basic principle is embedded within various teaching and learning methods and is commonly used by those who teach in veterinary skills labs. For instance, the four-step approach promoted by Walker and Peyton (1998) can be slightly modified and used in PAL courses (Krautter et al., 2011) (see Figure 8.1).

According to Nikendei et al. (2014), such a modification of the Peyton approach is particularly suitable for the instruction of small groups, which typically occurs in a clinical skills lab. The tutor first performs the exercise without any explanation ("demonstration"). In the next step, the tutor repeats the activity more slowly, explaining the steps ("deconstruction"). Afterwards, the tutee explains the action and the tutor executes it based on the instructions ("comprehension") of the tutee. For this step, the tutee has to understand the action and to reflect, recognize his or her own deficiencies, ask the tutor for clarification, and repeat again. At the end, the tutee carries out the exercise independently ("performance") and performs the skill.

Another similar method for teaching psychomotor skills is the five-step model according to George and Doto (2001) (see Chapter 3). Both methods can be used to teach a variety of clinical skills. In PAL courses, these methods are sometimes combined or slightly modified so that the learning outcomes of a specific clinical skill can be achieved.

When to Use PAL

There is potential for PAL to be used for a variety of clinical skills. Bates et al. (2016) describe a program between fifth (final) year and fourth year veterinary students, including canine clinical examination, suturing, bovine jugular

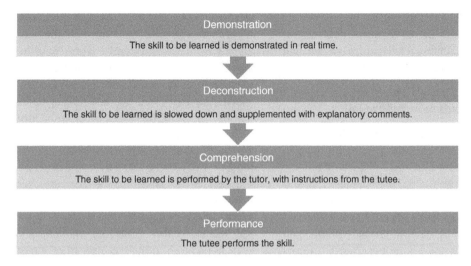

Figure 8.1 Modified version of Walker and Peyton's four-step-approach.

venipuncture, and bovine intramuscular injection. Third-year veterinary students taught students in the same year bovine rectal palpation via the use of a haptic simulator (Baillie et al., 2009). A medical student PAL program for clinical skills included measuring blood pressure, blood sampling, intravenous catheterization, and intramuscular injections (Weyrich et al., 2008). More broadly, PAL has also been used to teach communication skills (Nestel and Kidd, 2005; Strand et al., 2013), anatomy (Krych et al., 2005), clinical reasoning (Seycomb, 2008), and to revise knowledge prior to examinations (Wadoodi and Crosby, 2002; Bates et al., 2016).

When considering whether or not to incorporate PAL into your clinical skills teaching program, it is necessary to decide whether it will be a core (compulsory) part of the curriculum or optional. Bell et al. (2017) described use a compulsory, integrated PAL program for veterinary students, involving fourth-year students teaching first-year students how to perform a canine clinical examination. The program aimed to provide all fourth-year students with the opportunity to practice teaching and gain the benefits associated with this while providing additional learning opportunities for the first-year students. Wadoodi and Crosby (2002) discussed how PAL is often used to review subjects previously taught, while Seycomb

(2008) discussed how PAL can decrease staff supervision of tasks as student confidence increases.

Bates et al. (2016) described an optional PAL program involving final (fifth)-year veterinary students teaching fourth-year veterinary students a variety of clinical skills. There, the program took place in the evening outside of timetabled teaching with the aim to provide additional learning opportunities for students. Alternatively, optional programs can take place within the timetable for interested students or can be optional for the tutees, but not the tutors (Nestel and Kidd, 2005; Baillie et al., 2009).

PAL has also been used in the assessment of clinical skills. Since the use of university staff is expensive, various studies have investigated whether trained student examiners can also provide adequate assessments (Koch, 2008; Melcher et al., 2016; Khan et al., 2017). They found that student examiners are suitable, cost-effective, and can be used for formative objective structured clinical examinations (OSCEs). For this purpose, the already-experienced PAL tutors are particularly suitable (Melcher et al., 2016) and the tutees' acceptance of the student examiners is high (Koch, 2008). The use of student examiners from higher semesters is recommended, although feedback that promotes learning can be provided by examiners from all levels of experience (Khan et al., 2017). In general, the factors that influence the quality of (peer) assessments are reliability, relationships, stakes, and equivalence (Norcini, 2003).

Which Students to Include in PAL

When designing PAL teaching, it is necessary to decide which cohorts of students will be involved. Tutors and tutees can be from the same cohort (traditional or "true PAL") or different cohorts (sometimes referred to as cross-cohort or near-peer-assisted learning). These two approaches have different benefits and limitations; while more experienced tutors may have more knowledge than those within the same cohort, cross-cohort PAL within the curriculum makes timetabling and logistics more difficult. Weyrich et al. (2008) describe how a cross-cohort PAL program was used to teach clinical skills to lower year medical students, because it was deemed that only more senior students would have the necessary clinical experience to teach the relevant skills. In contrast, Baillie et al. (2009) initiated a program within the same cohort, with ease of organization stated as the primary reason for this choice.

In non-compulsory PAL programs, consideration needs to be given to how tutors will be recruited. While some programs recruit tutors based on academic ability (Ross and Cameron, 2007), Wadoodi and Crosby (2002) recommend that the opportunity to be a tutor should be given to all students within the relevant cohort. PAL is considered to be as beneficial for the tutor as for the tutee (see "Benefits for student tutor") so allowing lower ability students to partake allows all students the opportunity to benefit from the teaching experience. Tutors with lower academic ability may also be better placed to identify and help with gaps in tutee knowledge and so increase the value for these students (Wadoodi and Crosby, 2002). Some programs include a recruitment process, for example Weyrich et al. (2008) describe a recruitment interview for a paid tutor PAL program, with

selection criteria including level of motivation and prior experience of teaching. Renumeration can be provided as an incentive when recruiting tutors, although this is more commonly provided, for example in the United States than the United Kingdom (Wadoodi and Crosby, 2002; Ross and Cameron, 2007). The benefits and limitations of this must be considered – while extrinsic reward in the form of money may attract more students, care must be taken to ensure these students still have suitable intrinsic motivation and desire to teach (Wadoodi and Crosby, 2002; Weyrich et al., 2008).

In voluntary PAL programs, thought also needs to be given to the recruitment of tutees. More commonly, PAL is offered to all tutees within the chosen academic cohort, but it is also possible to offer to specific groups, for example lower achieving students (Wadoodi and Crosby, 2002; Ross and Cameron, 2007). As it is also a consideration for tutors, the motivation of the tutee to be involved needs to be considered. Tutees should be made aware of aims of the program and time commitment in advance, so they can decide whether the program is suitable for them (Wadoodi and Crosby, 2002).

For both tutors and tutees, care must be taken in the advertisement of voluntary PAL initiatives in order to ensure that all potential students are aware. It is important that advertisement does not inadvertently select against certain learners, for example those that do not read notice boards (Ross and Cameron, 2007). Some programs sent an email to all potential students, emphasizing that anyone could participate, while others described the project during a lecture period (Nestel and Kidd, 2005; Burgess et al., 2012; Bates et al., 2016).

A good PAL program will also be able to deal with excess demand for tutors and/or tutees. If a voluntary initiative is unable to accommodate all potential students, it is necessary to have a fair system for selecting individuals. This is particularly the case for tutees, where sign up rates may be high (Ross and Cameron, 2007). In initiatives with no selection criteria, some PAL programs operate on a "first come, first served" sign-up policy, while others randomly select participants based on those who are interested (Baillie et al., 2009; Bates et al., 2016).

Tutor Training

There is little to no consensus on the optimal training and education of tutors, although various studies have proven that training is a necessity (Kassab et al., 2005; Alvarez et al., 2017; van der Vleuten et al., 2017). Many studies describe an overall positive effect for the student tutors themselves as a result of tutor training (Nestel and Kidd, 2005; Blatt and Greenberg, 2007; Wong et al., 2007; Peets et al., 2009).

The goals of tutor training include achieving an equal level in knowledge, understanding, and skills of all tutors of the PAL initiative. There are two aspects to this – training in the skill in which they will be teaching, and training in how to lead and teach a session. The training that tutors require in the skill will vary depending on the aims and structure of the clinical skills program; however, at the end of the training session(s), each tutor should be able to design a lesson and teach a clinical skill to tutees in a structured way.

Topics for tutor training could include planning the session, setting the scene, writing objectives (learning outcomes), selecting a teaching approach (e.g. Peyton's four-step model; George and Doto's five-step model), closing the learning session, questioning the learner, and giving feedback (see Figure 8.2). In addition to the training, it is recommended that tutors be assigned to a specific set of skills that they will teach during the semester. This makes it easier for the tutor to establish a routine for the teaching. It can help tutors to write guidelines or manuals describing the clinical procedure and context of the skills within their teaching session. This is helpful for the tutors themselves, for other tutors (who may be teaching the same skill), and for quality management. For example, the manual can contain information about the equipment required, the scenario, the context, practical considerations, tasks for the tutees, a detailed description of the procedure (including photos or videos), references, and further readings. To ensure the clinical skill is taught correctly, the manuals should be reviewed by staff responsible for the clinical skill or teaching.

Helpful Strategies

Each PAL initiative will be different, depending on its aims and objectives, and this will influence how it is run. However, there are some general strategies that can help make any PAL program successful.

Wadoodi and Crosby (2002) describe how tutors in PAL prefer a certain amount of structure, but that this should not be so strict as to limit opportunities for discussion between tutors and tutees. The nature of this structure varies between PAL initiatives, but it is recommended to include support regarding what to cover and/or how. In a PAL program in which fourth-year veterinary students taught first-year veterinary students how to perform a clinical examination, tutors were provided with learning objectives on which the session must be based (Bell et al., 2017). These learning objectives had already been formally taught in the curriculum, so tutors could deliver these in any way in which they chose (Bell et al., 2017). A similar program by Bates et al. (2016) involved tutors teaching clinical skills already taught in the formal curriculum and required tutors to provide a lesson plan to be checked by staff. This plan had to follow a set format, as taught in the tutor training. Other PAL initiatives describe how students lead preplanned sessions; for example, Nestel and Kidd (2005) used student tutors to facilitate communication teaching in a pre-determined format. However, despite this stipulated format, tutors could still vary the way in which they gave information, meaning the session maintained the benefits of PAL. Weyrich et al. (2008) described a program with a high level of structure in which tutors teaching clinical skills to lower-year students were instructed to follow a tutor manual to ensure teaching was consistent.

Sections	Content
Planning the session	✓ Motivation ✓ Context of the skill in veterinary practice ✓ Background & knowledge of the tutees ✓ Learning objectives ✓ ...
Setting the scene	✓ Check the material (simulators, projection facilities, etc.) ✓ Adjust environment ✓ Check for time and schedule ✓ ...
Delivery	✓ Walker and Peyton's 5-step approach (1998) ✓ George and Doto's 4-step approach (2001) ✓ ...
Closure of the session	✓ Summarize ✓ Relation from start to end of the session ✓ Achievements ✓ ...
Feedback	✓ Self-reflection ✓ Positive feedback from the tutor ✓ Tips to perform better the next time ✓ ...

Figure 8.2 Example of possible sections and content for tutor training.

One of the benefits of PAL is that it often allows smaller group sizes compared to teaching by staff in the formal curriculum (see "Benefits for student tutees"), and so this must be considered when introducing a PAL initiative. Dubrowski and MacRae (2006) state that a ratio of one tutor to four tutees is optimal when teaching technical practical skills. In line with this recommendation, a ratio of one tutor to three or four tutees is often cited (Nestel and Kidd, 2005; Ross and Cameron, 2007; Weyrich et al., 2008; Baillie et al., 2009; Bates et al., 2016). In some initiatives, this is kept as one tutor to three or four tutees (Baillie et al., 2009), while in others, groups are combined to have two tutors for six to eight tutees (Nestel and Kidd, 2005; Weyrich et al., 2008; Bates et al., 2016).

One of the benefits of PAL is the safe atmosphere for learning. While this is created in part by using students as teachers, the environment in which the teaching takes place should also be considered. Wadoodi and Crosby (2002) recommend taking care when choosing a location and avoiding areas and resources that will encourage defaulting back to didactic teaching

(e.g. scheduling in lecture theatres, using PowerPoint presentations). Some initiatives provide food to help create a more informal atmosphere (Ross and Cameron, 2007).

Considerations

There are a number of limitations to PAL, as described above, but these can be minimized with careful planning.

The level of tutor knowledge is mentioned as a limitation of PAL by tutors, tutees, and staff. There are several ways to address this. Tutor training is naturally important; Weyrich et al. (2008) describe how fourth-year students received extra training in performing the clinical skills they were to teach. When the subject to be taught is novel to the tutors, for example bovine rectal palpation via use of a simulator (Baillie et al., 2009), all tutors were observed teaching at least one session by a member of staff. Ross and Cameron (2007) recommend considering tutors being in pairs when teaching as this can decrease the chance of erroneous teaching, while potentially allowing tutors to learn from each other.

When appropriate, Wadoodi and Crosby (2002) suggest rotating tutees between tutors for different activities, so tutees get exposed to tutors with different levels of knowledge. Choosing the appropriate cohort of tutors is also important; some programs select based on academic ability (Ross and Cameron, 2007), while others say this is not necessary providing tutors are encouraged to be honest with tutees about their level of knowledge (Wadoodi and Crosby, 2002).

Another commonly cited limitation of PAL is the ability of the tutor to teach. As for tutor knowledge, this can largely be tackled by appropriate training, as discussed in "Tutor training." In addition to training, some programs include prior experience of teaching as part of the selection process (Weyrich et al., 2008). For quality control of teaching standards, Baillie et al. (2009) describe how all tutors were observed teaching at least one session.

When initiating PAL, consideration must be given to the logistics and timetabling involved. Ross and Cameron (2007) maintain that this should not be a major problem long term if a program is set up well, but needs to be considered initially. Bell et al. (2017) recommend having well-defined plans that can be followed each year with one individual responsible for overseeing all organization. A guide for running PAL has been created to aid handover between cohorts of students, and this is freely available online (Bates and Baillie, 2016). For PAL courses within a curriculum, timetabling can be problematic and needs to be approached long in advance (Bell et al., 2017) but is easier to manage if tutors and tutees are within the same cohort (Baillie et al., 2009).

Finally, it can be worth considering having a staff member present but out of sight. This can benefit deficits in tutor knowledge, tutor teaching ability, and help with logistics. For example, Ross and Cameron (2007) had a member of staff present to help with organization at the beginning of the session and available throughout in case of needle-stick injury. Bates et al. (2016) describe how a member of staff was present but not involved, and Krych et al. (2005) had a teaching assistant available as a "resource" in case needed. In a program involving senior medical students teaching clinical skills to lower-year students, tutors appreciated having a member of staff available for questions if necessary (Weyrich et al., 2008). If staff are present, their input should be minimal to encourage the safe atmosphere that benefits PAL (Wadoodi and Crosby, 2002).

Conclusions

The process of students teaching other students, known as peer-assisted learning or PAL, has been used to successfully teach clinical skills in a variety of medical and veterinary disciplines. PAL can benefit the student who is teaching (tutor), the student who is learning (tutee), and the institution itself, with only a small number of manageable limitations. The teaching of clinical skills via PAL can be incorporated into the curriculum as a compulsory activity or be an option. It can include students within the same year or across different cohorts. Regardless of how it will be delivered, it is important to train the tutors, and it can be helpful to provide structure for the session, to keep group sizes small and to encourage an informal atmosphere. Finally, to minimize the impact of any potential limitations, consideration must be given to the level of tutor knowledge, teaching ability, and the initial planning and logistics involved.

References

Aburahma, M. H., Mohamed, H. M. 2017. Peer teaching as an educational tool in pharmacy schools; fruitful or futile. *Curr Pharm Teach Learn*, 9, 1170–1179.

Agius, A., Calleja, N., Camenzuli, C., et al. 2018. Perceptions of first-year medical students towards learning anatomy using cadaveric specimens through peer teaching. *Anat Sci Educ*, 11, 346–357.

Alvarez, S., Dethleffsen, K., Esper, T., et al. 2017. An overview of peer tutor training strategies at German medical schools. *Z Evid Fortbild Qual Gesundhwes*, 126, 77–83.

Amorosa, J. M. H., Mellman L. A., Graham, M. J. 2011. Medical students as teachers: How preclinical teaching opportunities can create an early awareness of the role of physician as teacher. *Med Teach*, 33, 137–144.

Baillie, S., Shore, H., Gill, D., et al. 2009. Introducing peer-assisted learning into a veterinary curriculum: A trial with a simulator. *J Vet Med Educ*, 36, 174–179.

Bates, L. S. W., Baillie, S. 2016. vetPAL Student Leader Handbook. http://www.bris.ac.uk/vetscience/media/docs/vetpalhandbook.pdf Accessed September 24, 2020.

Bates, L. S. W., Warman, S., Pither, Z., et al. 2016. Development and evaluation of vetPAL, a student-led, peer-assisted learning program. *J Vet Med Educ*, 43, 382–389.

Bell, C. E., Rhind, S. M., Stansbie, N. H., et al. 2017. Getting started with peer-assisted learning in a veterinary curriculum. *J Vet Med Educ*, 44, 640–648.

Benè, K. L., Bergus, G. 2014. When learners become teachers. *Fam Med*, 46, 783–787.

Blatt, B., Greenberg, L. 2007. A multi-level assessment of a program to teach medical students to teach. *Adv Health Sci Educ Theory Pract*, 12, 7–18.

Brueckner, J. K., MacPherson, B. R. 2004. Benefits from peer teaching in the dental gross anatomy laboratory. *Eur J Dent Educ*, 8, 72–77.

Bulte, C., Betts, A., Garner, K., et al. 2007. Student teaching: Views of student near-peer teachers and learners. *Med Teach*, 29, 583–590.

Burgess, A., Black, K., Chapman, E., et al. 2012. Teaching skills for students: Our future educators. *Clin Teach*, 9, 312–316.

Dandavino, M., Snell, L., Wiseman, J. 2007. Why medical students should learn how to teach. *Med Teach*, 29, 558–565.

Devin-Sheehan, L., Feldman, R. S., Allen, V. L. 1976. Research on children tutoring children: A critical review. *Rev Educ Res*, 46, 355–385.

Dubrowski, A., MacRae, H. 2006. Randomised, controlled study investigating the optimal instructor: Student ratios for teaching suturing skills. *Med Educ*, 40, 59–63.

Engelskirchen, S., Ehlers, J., Kirk, A. T., et al. 2017. Skills lab training in veterinary medicine. Effective preparation for clinical work at the small animal clinic of the University for Veterinary Medicine Hannover, Foundation. *Tierarztliche Praxis. Ausgabe K, Kleintiere/Heimtiere*, 45 (06): 397–405.

Evans, D. J., Cuffe, T. 2009. Near-peer teaching in anatomy: An approach for deeper learning. *Anat Sci Educ*, 2, 227–233.

Fantuzzo, J. W., Riggio, R. E., Connelly, S., et al. 1989. Effects of reciprocal peer tutoring on academic achievement and psychological adjustment: A component analysis. *J Educ Psychol* 81, 173–177.

Fincher, R., Simpson, D., Mennin, S., et al. 2000. Scholarship in teaching: an imperative for the 21st century. *Acad Med*, 75, 887–894.

George, J. H., Doto, F. X. 2001. A simple five-step method for teaching clinical skills. *Fam Med*, 33, 577–578.

GMC. 2018. Outcomes for Graduates 2018. https://www.gmc-uk.org/-/media/documents/dc11326-outcomes-for-graduates-2018_pdf-75040796.pdf Accessed June 2, 2021.

Goldschmid, B., Goldschmid, L. M. 1976. Peer teaching in higher education: A review. *High Educ*, 5, 9–33.

Hammond, J. A., Bithell, C. P., Jones, L., et al. 2010. A first year experience of student-directed peer-assisted learning. *Active Learn High Educ* 11, 201–212.

Issenberg, B. S., McGaghie, W. C., Petrusa, E. R. et al. 2005. Features and uses of high-fidelity medical simulations that lead to effective learning: a BEME systematic review. *Med Teach*, 27, 10–28.

Kassab, S., Abu-Hijleh, M. F., Al-Shboul, Q., et al. 2005. Student-led tutorials in problem-based learning: Educational outcomes and students' perceptions. *Med Teach*, 27, 521–526.

Khan, R., Payne, M. W., Chahine, S. 2017. Peer assessment in the objective structured clinical examination: a scoping review. *Med Teach*, 39, 745–756.

Koch, A. 2008. Studentische Tutoren als Prüfer in einer"objective structured clinical examination"(OSCE): Evaluation ihrer Bewertungsleistungen (Doctoral dissertation, Niedersächsische Staats-und Universitätsbibliothek Göttingen).

Krautter, M., Weyrich, P., Schultz, J. H., et al. 2011. Effects of Peyton's four-step approach on objective performance measures in technical skills training: A controlled trial. *Teach Learn Med*, 23, 244–250.

Krych, A. J., March, C. N., Bryan, R. E., et al. 2005. Reciprocal peer teaching: Students teaching students in gross anatomy laboratory. *Med Educ*, 18, 261–301.

Lockspeiser, T. M., O'Sullivan, P., Teherani, A., et al. 2008. Understanding the experience of being taught by peers: the value of social and cognitive congruence. *Adv Health Sci Educ*, 13, 361–372.

McWhorter, D. L., Forester, J. P. 2004. Effects of an alternate dissection schedule on gross anatomy laboratory practical performance. *Clin Anat*, 17, 144–148.

Melcher, P., Zajonz, D., Roth, A., et al. 2016. Peer-assisted teaching student tutors as examiners in an orthopedic surgery OSCE station–pros and cons. *GMS Interdiscip Plast Reconstr Surg DGPW*, 5, Doc 17.

Michaelsen, L. K., Sweet, M. 2011. Team-based learning. *New Dir Teach Learn*, 2011, 128, 41–51.

Monahan, C. M., Yew, A. C. 2002. Adapting a case-based, cooperative learning strategy to a veterinary parasitology laboratory. *J Vet Med Educ*, 29, 186–192.

Morris, D., Turnbull, P. 2004. Using student nurses as teachers in inquiry-based learning. *J Adv Nurs*, 45, 136–144.

Nestel, D., Kidd, J. 2005. Peer assisted learning in patient-centred interviewing: The impact on student tutors. *Med Teach*, 27, 439–444.

Nikendei, C., Huber, J., Stiepak, J., et al. 2014. Modification of Peyton's four-step approach for small group teaching - a descriptive study. *BMC Med Educ*, 14, 68.

Norcini, J. J. 2003. Peer assessment of competence. *Med Educ*, 37, 539–543.

Peets, A.D., Coderre, S., Wright, B., et al. 2009. Involvement in teaching improves learning in medical students: a randomised cross-over study. *BMC Med Educ*, 9, 55.

Royal College of Veterinary Surgeons. 2020. Day One Competences. https://www.rcvs.org.uk/document-library/day-one-competences/ Accessed May 28, 2021.

Ross, M. T., Cameron, H. S. 2007. Peer assisted learning: a planning and implementation framework: AMEE guide no. 30. *Med Teach*, 27, 527–545.

Schmidt, H. G., Moust, J. H. C. 1995. What makes a tutor effective? A structural-equations modeling approach to learning in problem-based curricula. *Acad Med*, 70, 708–714.

Schnabel, K. P., Boldt, P. D., Breuer, G., et al. 2011. A consensus statement on practical skills in medical school – a position paper by the GMA committee on practical skills. *GMS Z Med Ausbild*, 28, Doc58.

Seenan, C., Shanmugam, S., Stewart, J. 2016. Group peer teaching: A strategy for building confidence in communication and teamwork skills in physical therapy students. *J Phys Ther Educ*, 30, 40–49.

Seycomb, J. 2008. A systematic review of peer teaching and learning in clinical education. *J Clin Nurs*, 17, 703–716.

Solomon, P., Crowe, J. 2001. Perceptions of student peer tutors in a problem-based learning programme. *Med Teach*, 23, 181–186.

Soriano, R. P., Blatt, B., Coplitt, L., et al. 2010. Teaching medical students how to teach: A national survey of students-as-teachers programs in U.S. medical schools. *Acad Med*, 85, 1725–1731.

Strand, E. B., Johnson, B., Thompson, J. 2013. Peer-assisted communication training: Veterinary students as simulated clients and communication skills trainers. *J Vet Med Educ*, 40, 233–241.

ten Cate, O. 2017. Perspective paper/perspektive: Peer teaching: From method to philosophy. *Zeitschrift für Evidenz, Fortbildung und Qualität im Gesundheitswesen*, 127, 85–87.

ten Cate, O., Durning, S. 2007a. Dimensions and psychology of peer teaching in medical education. *Med Teach*, 29, 546–552.

ten Cate, O., Durning, S. 2007b. Peer teaching in medical education: Twelve reasons to move from theory to practice. *Med Teach*, 29, 591–599.

Tolsgaard, M. G., Gustafsson, A., Rasmussen, M. B., et al. 2007. Student teachers can be as good as associate professors in teaching clinical skills. *Med Teach*, 29, 553–557.

Topping, K. J. 1996. The effectiveness of peer tutoring in further and higher education: A typology and review of the literature. *High Educ*, 32, 321–345.

Topping, K. J. 2005. Trends in peer learning. *Educ Psychol*, 25, 631–345.

Topping, K. J., Ehly, S. W. 2001. Peer assisted learning: A framework for consultation. *J Educ Psychol Consult*, 12, 113–132.

van der Vleuten, C., Sluijsman, D., Joosten-ten Brinke, D. 2017. Competence assessment as learner support in education. In: *Competence-Based Vocational and Professional Education*. Mulder, M. (ed.) Cham: Springer, pp. 607–630.

Wadoodi, A., Crosby, J. R. 2002. Twelve tips for peer-assisted learning: a classic concept revisited. *Med Teach*, 24, 241–244.

Walker, M., Peyton, J. W. R. 1998. Teaching in the theatre. In: *Teaching and Learning in Medical Practice*. Peyton, J. W. R. (ed.) Rickmansworth: Manticore Publishers Europe Ltd, pp. 171–180.

Weyrich, P., Schrauth, M., Kraus, B., et al. 2008. Undergraduate technical skills training guided by student tutors – analysis of tutors' attitudes, tutees' acceptance and learning progress in an innovative teaching model. *BMC Med Educ*, 8, 18.

Wong, J. G., Waldrep, T. D., Smith, T. G. 2007. Formal peer-teaching in medical school improves academic performance: The MUSC supplemental instructor program. *Teach Learn Med*, 19, 216–220.

Yu, T., Wilson, N. C., Singh, P. P., et al. 2011. Medical students-as-teachers: A systematic review of peer-assisted teaching during medical school. *Adv Med Educ Pract*, 2, 157–172.

Zentz, S. E., Kurtz, C. P., Alverson, E. M. 2014. Undergraduate peer-assisted learning in the clinical setting. *J Nurs Educ*, 53, 4–10.

9

What Other Skills Are Vital to Successful Clinical Practice?

Elizabeth Armitage-Chan[1] and Susan M. Matthew[2]

[1] *LIVE Centre, Department of Clinical Sciences and Services, Royal Veterinary College, Hatfield, UK*
[2] *Department of Veterinary Clinical Sciences, College of Veterinary Medicine, Washington State University, Pullman, WA, USA*

Key Messages

- Being an effective and successful practitioner involves many skills beyond those of technical performance
- Being able to discuss clinical treatment plans with clients and individualize decision-making according to varying client and patient needs is essential
- Collaboration and high-quality communication enhance clinical care and ensure that both client and veterinarian are active participants in clinical decision-making
- Effective management of challenging situations that arise from influences beyond the complexity of the clinical disease is important for resilience, well-being, and career satisfaction and longevity

---

Introduction

Being a good veterinarian involves integrating many different competencies at the same time. Furthermore, an individual's idea of a "good veterinarian" may not be the same as everyone else's. While previous chapters in this book have examined the teaching, learning, and assessment of clinical skills and associated knowledge, this chapter looks specifically at additional competencies that enable veterinarians to effectively practice.

Being a veterinarian involves diagnosing and treating disease, but this process is invariably influenced by broader complicating factors: the financial resources that are available to the client, the needs of the client and their beliefs about animal care, differing opinions among colleagues as to the "right" way to manage a particular disease, etc. The skills discussed in this chapter are intended to enhance problem-solving and decision-making in situations that commonly arise, many of which are characterized by uncertainty and ambiguity, where there is a lack of assurance that the chosen action will lead to a desirable outcome. Being competent at managing such situations, and analyzing and learning from them, is key to developing resilience to the many challenges of veterinary practice. Through the application of advanced collaboration, communication, conflict resolution, and teamwork skills, a veterinarian is better

Veterinary Clinical Skills, First Edition. Edited by Emma K. Read, Matt R. Read, and Sarah Baillie.
© 2022 John Wiley & Sons, Inc. Published 2022 by John Wiley & Sons, Inc.
Companion website: www.wiley.com/go/read/veterinary

placed to achieve more desirable outcomes that truly reflect the wishes of all the participants involved.

Scenarios like the one described in Box 9.1 are all too common across all areas of clinical veterinary practice. Becoming proficient in the skills required to resolve this type of situation is essential for achieving success as a veterinarian. Clinical reasoning may direct the veterinarian toward several different options in each case: diagnostic tests to run, presumptive diagnoses to act on, symptomatic care to provide, or curative treatments to offer. Each part of the plan will have benefits for some of the stakeholders, but some might not suit the priorities of all involved. The veterinarian often will not know which route will yield the best outcome for all, with even "gold standard" management carrying risks of error (e.g. incorrect diagnosis) or failure (e.g. lack of response to treatment). Working with all of this uncertainty can be challenging, let alone when these cases are also accompanied by aspects of communication, negotiation, financial responsibility, client care, and self-management.

The concept of "gold standard" care involves arriving at a definitive diagnosis and implementing the treatment associated with the greatest likelihood of disease resolution. However, in many situations the gold standard might involve temporary welfare compromise for the patient or be simply unachievable for the client (Grimm et al., 2018). Not being able to implement the gold standard approach that was taught in veterinary school has been proposed as a contributor to poor mental health in the profession, because highly academic, hard-working and perfectionist-prone graduates see this care as the standard of being a "good veterinarian" (Armitage-Chan and May, 2018; Armitage-Chan, 2019a). Anything that prevents diagnosis and treatment, such as a client with limited resources, can often be seen as obstructive to individual professional priorities and act as a source of frustration and career distress.

For veterinarians, the way they define success in practice and what it actually means to be an excellent veterinarian can represent an important part of their professional identity. Research has found that veterinarians who possess an

---

Box 9.1   Example of a Common Situation in Clinical Practice

Scenario: The Sick Puppy

It is your first month in practice and your first Saturday in sole charge of the clinic. A client arrives with a six-month-old puppy that started vomiting this morning. You are fairly sure the puppy has an easily treatable problem. You recommend some symptomatic treatment and then further diagnostics. The client starts crying, then explains that they have no money and asks you if you can reduce their costs. You agree to start supportive care for the puppy while the client goes home to discuss finances with their family. Two hours later the client's partner calls you on the telephone. They angrily accuse you of only caring about money and insist that the puppy be euthanized immediately. You speak to the client who states that they cannot accept this course of action, nor will they consent to rehoming the puppy.

What action do you take now? Proceed with treatment along the intention of reducing the costs or suggest a payment plan that might make care more affordable? Become frustrated that people cannot pay for the needs of their pet? Try to convince the client to consent to the proposed diagnostic and treatment plan as is? Euthanize the puppy? Or apply your skills in communication, collaboration, client care, and shared decision-making to negotiate a new plan that, while not being perfect, is acceptable to all?

identity centered exclusively around clinical diagnosis and treatment tend to resent contextual challenges to their clinical plans, such as those caused by a clients' limited financial resources or differing beliefs about animal care. These veterinarians can easily become frustrated and disaffected by their work as a result of this disconnect (Armitage-Chan and May, 2018). In contrast, those who experience a sense of success from working through difficult decisions with clients tend to more effectively integrate these challenges into their professional identity and experience a greater sense of satisfaction with their daily work. These veterinarians tend to place increased value on both their clinical skills and on competencies associated with client negotiation and collaboration, viewing them as essential for their long-term success in practice. In contrast, veterinarians who prioritize clinical diagnosis and treatment tend to see communication skills as a tool that is applied to educate or persuade the client to agree with the veterinarian's preferred clinical plan.

Decision-Making in Situations of Complexity and Uncertainty

Veterinarians often need to make decisions in practice without knowing for certain the best action that will yield the most successful patient management or the most optimal outcome for the client. Questioning clients about what they value most in their veterinarian reveals their belief that veterinarians can be all things to all people: clinically skilled and knowledgeable, able to empathize with and incorporate each clients' individual needs, able to communicate clearly (particularly when the client is stressed or overwhelmed by the situation), and animal-oriented (able to care for animals, prioritize their welfare and be skilled in low stress handling) (Gregório et al., 2016; Hughes et al., 2018). It is thus hardly surprising that being able to meet client expectations is one of the most frequently described career stressors (Gardner and Hini, 2006). Managing clients' varied needs, as well as running a business, makes decision-making in practice highly complex.

In the scenario at the start of this chapter (Box 9.1), the veterinarian could use the information that they obtained from the history and physical examination to make an "educated best guess" that the puppy is experiencing a simple case of dietary indiscretion. In view of the client's situation, the veterinarian might recommend that 12 hours of intravenous fluid administration will help the pup's dehydration and withholding food for 24 hours will likely cause the vomiting to subside, resulting in recovery without requiring further tests to confirm the presumptive diagnosis. In most presented cases, the veterinarian's plan would be effective; it will not cost the client a lot of money, the puppy will feel better once it is rehydrated, and there will be no compromise in case outcome. However, there remains a small risk that gastrointestinal obstruction or some other pathology may be present, which might not be detected without additional diagnostic testing. The fluid therapy could therefore constitute "wasted" time if the puppy were to eventually need further tests or if the puppy should have been euthanized initially. The veterinarian's initial decision was an educated choice, but that does not necessarily mean that success is guaranteed.

Managing financial limitations of the client is a particularly common and high-stakes contributor to uncertainty in decision-making and is one of the most significant stresses facing veterinarians (Batchelor and McKeegan, 2012; Platt et al., 2012; Kipperman et al., 2017). From the client's viewpoint, openly discussing the financial implications of any chosen treatment, as well as being able to balance pet care decisions, is an essential veterinary skill (Coe et al., 2007). Many clients report that they want their financial limitations considered during clinical decision-making; however, the reality is that they are also reluctant to concede that their own financial limitations might take precedence over the quality of veterinary care that can be provided (Coe et al., 2007; Hughes et al., 2018). This tension between what they want and what they can afford means that factoring in a client's financial limitations when making clinical decisions is highly complex, and very common. The high prevalence of financial concerns among veterinary clients (Volk et al., 2011), the detrimental impact of client resource limitations on veterinarians' stress and career satisfaction (Kipperman et al., 2017) and the lack of attention to frank cost discussions with clients (Coe et al., 2009), all suggest that handling financial tensions is one of the most important skills of the successful clinician.

Ethical dilemmas are also a common part of everyday veterinary practice. They inevitably invoke uncertainty and contribute to stress because they cause deviation from linear, predictable problem-solving, creating obstacles for preferred clinical actions (e.g. financial limitations, client preferences), and cause requests from clients or colleagues to pursue actions with which the veterinarian disagrees (Batchelor and McKeegan, 2012; Moses et al. 2018). The need to act in the face of uncertainty conflicts with the need for perfectionism by many veterinarians, thus further contributing to anxiety and distress (Clarke and Knights, 2018).

Veterinarians faced with these types of dilemmas often have numerous possible options or solutions available, none of which may feel ideal. A systematic approach can help to manage complex, uncertain decisions and ensures that the risks and benefits of various alternatives have been fully considered.

One effective problem-solving approach that can be used is based on a framework for systematic ethical reasoning (Armitage-Chan, 2019b). The first step is to identify all of the options available for solving the problem, including those that the veterinarian might initially feel are inappropriate or suboptimal. Once the veterinarian has identified all the options they can possibly think of, they can then analyze them for strengths and weaknesses according to the needs and priorities of all the stakeholders who will be affected by their decision. This process includes considering what needs to be achieved for each factor (e.g. a baseline acceptable level of animal welfare; avoiding options that would put the client

into unacceptable levels of debt) and what is desirable (e.g. the patient being able to return home). Integrating immediate considerations (e.g. attending to animal welfare, supporting the client's attachment to their pet) with longer term and broader ones (e.g. the long-time financial implications for the client, retaining a long-term relationship with the client, supporting a positive reputation for the veterinary practice) help ensure that the veterinarian assesses each option fully and rigorously. The eventual decision that the veterinarian makes, achieved through collaborative communication with the client, is well-informed and is based on the advantages and benefits to patient care, as well as the potential risks or complications to the client and veterinarian. This helps avoid risk and minimizes the impact of negative outcomes.

Communication

Effective communication skills are vital for successful clinical consultations and for productive workplace communications. Fortunately, the ability to communicate effectively is not an inherent attribute that you are necessarily born with. Instead, it is a series of learned skills that may be developed through deliberate practice: critically reflecting on an experience or incident to identify lapses and challenges, goal-setting to define areas for improvement (such as managing emotional or highly-charged conversations), requesting and reflecting upon feedback (which, after graduating from the formal education environment of the university, may come from clients or colleagues) and accessing resources such as published literature or continuing education sessions that inform personal development in areas such as communication skills, self-awareness, etc. (Ericsson, 2004).

Several models have been developed that highlight different aspects of communication and relationship-building during the veterinary clinical consultation (Shaw, 2006; Adams and Frankel, 2007; Cornell and Kopcha, 2007). These frameworks provide an excellent basis from which communication can be analyzed and developed through critical reflection. One of the most detailed models available is the Calgary-Cambridge Guide to the Clinical Consultation (Silverman et al., 2005), which has been more recently contextualized to veterinary medicine (Adams and Kurtz, 2017). Together the stages and processes of the Calgary-Cambridge Model are 71 discrete skills, which may be drawn upon and practiced to improve performance (Silverman et al., 2005; Adams and Kurtz, 2017).

The clinical consultation models described above all highlight the importance of rapport building and attention to relational conversation elements just as much as to clinical information. As new graduate veterinarians develop their communication skills, they become highly competent in effectively managing the clinical elements of conversations, for example history-taking and discussing animal health. However, the types of emotionally charged conversations that are implicit in the case example (Box 9.1) at the start of this chapter will always remain more challenging. Deliberate practice to improve clinical communication skills will therefore involve identifying challenges (communicating effectively in heightened emotions) and goals (improving conversation management in such contexts). Using clinical consultation models can be helpful to reflectively analyze client interactions to highlight an absence of rapport or relationship building, demonstrate a dominance of clinical-factual content rather than emphasis on relational elements, or suggest a need for greater focus on empathy or elements of emotional intelligence (e.g. self-awareness, self-management, social awareness, or relationship management) (Mayer and Salovey, 1997; Goleman, 1998; Goleman et al., 2002; Freedman, 2007).

The stages and processes within the Calgary-Cambridge model may help to inform improvement. Where decision-making is complex and may be confusing for the client, this model is useful to highlight the importance of preparing the client for decision-making, gather information about the client's understanding of the situation (as well as their needs and desire for a successful outcome), provide structure through signposting the elements of the decision-making process and checking the client's understanding of complicated information, and relationship building (e.g. focusing on client care, empathy, and attention to the client's needs).

Collaboration

Effectively working with clients and others – especially in challenging situations – involves both communication skills and an understanding of human interactions and responses. The aim of collaboration is to achieve a mutually reached and shared decision, one that is achieved neither through simply persuading the client to engage in the veterinarian's preferred plan nor by placing responsibility for decision-making solely on the client. Instead, by working to understand the client's perspective, the veterinarian can individualize their guidance and recommendations, tailoring both to ensure that patient welfare needs, practice business interests, and personal values are all met. Communication is therefore focused less on informing and persuading the client, and more on fostering a collaborative partnership for problem-solving (Silverman et al., 2005; Cornell and Kopcha, 2007; Adams and Kurtz, 2017).

This collaborative partnership requires empathy, so that the veterinarian is able to fully understand and address their client's needs, and high-quality communication to create the trust required for the client to discuss their values and priorities with the veterinarian (Silverman et al., 2005; Shaw, 2006). In the presence of a critically ill pet, high economic costs, or fears of bereavement, communication will be challenged by the tension of conflicting needs and the impact of heightened emotions. Emotional intelligence, including self-awareness, is needed to identify the veterinarian's own contributions to the quality of the communication, such as realizing when they are becoming frustrated or defensive and the impact this emotional response is likely to have on the conversation (Goleman et al., 2002).

Effective collaboration with clients in difficult situations involves more than simply applying communication models. There is significant overlap with ethics, incorporating a need to understand and authentically empathize, with a different set of goals and priorities to one's own. Ethical reasoning describes the systematic analysis of ethical dilemmas to appreciate the needs and perspectives of all stakeholders (Mullan and Main, 2001). Communication models such as those described above are applied with the aim of gathering information about the client's needs, validating their viewpoints, and actively enquiring about and engaging with the client's perspective. The integration of ethical and communication competencies thus supports collaborative client interactions and shared problem-solving. Ethics and communication are applied in parallel, enhancing empathy, relationship building, and interpersonal interaction. Therefore, we encourage veterinarians to reflect both on their communication skills, and also on the strategies they use to understand and empathize with clients' perspectives. Strategies such as asking open-ended questions, then providing time for clients to process the situation and explain their concerns, become methods by which the veterinarian can better understand and incorporate the client's viewpoint.

How is collaboration achieved? The essence of a collaborative partnership is that it is *two-way*: communication passes from the client to the veterinarian and the veterinarian to the client in equal measure. Focusing on collaboration, as described above, rather than *one-way* communication (that is intended to direct or persuade the client to the veterinarian's preferred action) means analyzing one's own influence within the conversation. Rather than simply focusing on whether the information provided is clearly and empathically delivered, the veterinarian considers the extent to which they invite the client to speak and whether they build trust, enabling the client to provide their views. The way a veterinarian responds could potentially inhibit the client from fully explaining their concerns. Collaboration will be fostered

more effectively by encouraging the client to embrace their role within the partnership. Active listening is a technique that encourages the client to talk, and hence to discuss their needs and their desired outcome (Robertson, 2005). Without actively trying to obtain their client's views, concerns, and needs relating to the case, it will be impossible for the veterinarian to incorporate the client's perspective when they make suggestions for clinical management. Emotional intelligence is required on the part of the veterinarian to analyze their own responses and body language, and evaluate whether they encourage or inhibit the client from telling their full story (Robertson, 2005). The same skills are equally relevant for interactions with coworkers and others.

Conflict Resolution

Communication, collaboration, and decision-making are particularly challenging when the priorities, values, and goals that contribute to a veterinarian's professional identity are in conflict with those of colleagues, or with the personal needs, values, and priorities held by the client. The Thomas-Kilman conflict resolution model states that conflict can be resolved using different strategies, which fall across a spectrum, based on the extent to which they involve *cooperativeness* (i.e. satisfying others' concerns) versus *assertiveness* (i.e. satisfying one's own concerns) (Thomas, 1992). A veterinarian might assume that their goal during conflict is to become more assertive to convince a client of the need to pursue the veterinarian's clinical recommendation. This course of action could be assumed both for the animal's sake, and because there is evidence of burnout among veterinarians demonstrating too little personal assertiveness with a feeling of constantly making decisions to appease the client (Moses et al., 2018). In a minority of situations, an animal's compromised welfare is so severe that actions such as euthanasia must be taken immediately, regardless of the client's wishes. It could be argued that in such situations, a clear and assertive approach is required. However, in their Code of Professional Conduct, the Royal College of Veterinary Surgeons (the British professional regulator) advises that such situations are very rare and that in cases of conflict between the needs of the patient and the needs of the client, the veterinarian should concentrate their efforts on working with the client to reach a mutually acceptable decision (RCVS, 2018). This process represents a collaborative approach to conflict management in which assertiveness and cooperativeness must be balanced (Thomas, 1992). The veterinarian should neither dismiss their concerns about the patient and recommendations for clinical management in favor of the client's wishes nor take the view that the only successful outcome occurs when the client's primary choice of patient care is implemented. In all but the most severely compromised patient welfare cases, symptomatic treatment can usually be given to alleviate pain and suffering during a process of negotiation, which may occur over a sustained period of time as a trusting, collaborative relationship is constructed.

Fostering positive relationships with clients provides significant career satisfaction (Armitage-Chan, 2019b). However, the nature of veterinary work means there will be many frequent situations where clients receive bad news, encounter significant financial costs, or face the imminent loss of their pet. It is therefore not to be expected that all veterinarian–client interactions will be positive. Feelings of anger will be common for both the veterinarian and client during situations that involve illness, death, and significant financial cost. This is because anger has many origins, including part of the grieving process, or when one is fearful, and when one's values are judged or questioned (Cerney and Buskirk, 1991; Philip et al., 2007). Being able to analyze the presence of anger (one's own, or that of the client) is part of the emotional intelligence required to manage difficult situations. Without being able to logically and systemically analyze the emotions present during a highly charged conversation, the interaction becomes reactive and intuitive rather than analytical and cognitive (Koole and Jostmann, 2004). When this happens in an interaction, the quality of the conversation will decline and the outcome is unlikely to be perceived as successful. Accepting that some clients are likely to be angry, processing this situation analytically and using the resulting understanding to empathize with the client rather than regard them as "difficult" represents part of the higher level, multifaceted process of effectively managing tension and interpersonal collaboration through emotional intelligence, as well as effective communication skills (Halpern, 2007).

Resilience

Veterinary students and veterinarians demonstrate a desire to be challenged in their work (Tomlin et al., 2010; Mastenbroek et al., 2014; Cake et al., 2015; Cake et al., 2019). However, the mental health literature identifies the most significant negative impact on veterinarians' wellbeing occurs when linear clinical reasoning – the pathway from presenting signs to diagnosis and treatment that is often modelled in university clinical teaching – is complicated by everyday challenges such as financial limitations or clients' belief systems that are oriented away from the importance of diagnosis and advanced treatments (Clarke and Knights, 2018). All veterinarians, whether they thrive in clinical practice or not, will encounter these challenges. Those who thrive are able to recognize that they are confronted by the difficult task of managing these "everyday challenges," but are confident that they possess the necessary competence to overcome them (e.g. the collaborative approach to communication and problem-solving described above). They also, most importantly, perceive this "in-the-moment problem-solving" to be an important and valuable skill (Cake et al., 2015). In particular, a distinction has been made between veterinarians who consider client-based challenges to be obstructive to their clinical plans, and those who see these challenges, and the competencies required to manage them, as integral to their veterinary work (Armitage-Chan and May, 2018).

The good news is that, like communication skills, resilience is not an attribute that a person either has or does not have (Mansfield et al., 2016; McArthur et al., 2017). Instead, resilience can be built by developing resources, both within and around yourself, and can be strengthened by implementing strategies to navigate the challenges that you will face in practice (Mansfield et al., 2016; McArthur et al., 2017).

A range of personal and contextual resources are helpful in building the capacity for resilience. Personal resources include emotional intelligence, motivation, optimism, and assertiveness (Ryan and Deci, 2000; Goleman et al., 2002; Seligman, 2006; Cake et al., 2017). Contextual resources include those available in the workplace that an individual personally fosters: colleagues and mentors; feedback on performance; and support from family and friends (Cake et al., 2017).

Many strategies can be used to enhance resilience. These strategies include nurturing one's personal life and relationships outside of work, engaging in professional development and reflective practice, drawing on professional counselling services when they might be helpful, and employing effective coping strategies such as problem-solving, humor, and reframing situations to view them differently (Carver, 1997; Cake et al., 2017; McArthur et al., 2019; Armitage-Chan, 2019a). Reframing situations is a useful skill that includes placing value on the enhanced veterinary care that can be provided by establishing positive client relationships. Drawing on these resources and strategies will help to create the outcome of resilience (Mansfield et al., 2016; McArthur et al., 2017), as well as the potential for increased well-being, engagement, and job satisfaction (Demerouti et al., 2001; Cake et al., 2017; Mastenbroek, 2017). While many veterinarians experience career stressors at some point, it has been shown they can be managed in such a way that they do not become overwhelming and lead to burnout or exhaustion (Cake et al., 2017; Moses et al., 2018; Arbe Montoya et al., 2019).

Teamwork

Veterinarians who thrive in the profession and appear resilient to its challenges describe the importance of maintaining positive relationships within their workplace team (Moore et al., 2014). Veterinarians' teamwork experience is unique, in that the "team" is often mostly absent: clinicians share cases with colleagues who they may rarely or never see, and many veterinarians work in small practices with few colleagues overall (Armitage-Chan et al., 2016). This situation can be particularly challenging for new graduate veterinarians when attempting to integrate into the team, since traditional approaches to fostering a positive team dynamic (e.g. such as socializing together or collaborating in clinical problem-solving) may not be feasible. However, the way the veterinary team operates, including how engaged the team members are and how they avoid creating a "toxic" team environment, contributes to the new graduate's job satisfaction and prevention of burnout (Moore et al., 2014). Teamworking skills are therefore both important in the provision of high-quality clinical practice and also in the support of positive individual well-being (Kinnison et al., 2015).

Veterinarians can help to create an effective team by contributing to a positive workplace culture that values both productivity and interpersonal relationships. Effective teamwork is built on fostering trust among team members and establishing a "no blame" culture where all team members are open to feedback focused on improving performance (Ruby and DeBowes, 2007; Lencioni, 2008; Viner, 2010). It also requires commitment by each team member to the practice's mission, in order to focus on creating successful outcomes for clients and patients, and to create accountability for individual and team performance. There are many teamwork models available, some of which are summarized by Moonaisur and Parumasur (2012). However, teamwork skills vary depending on the task: those skills required for managing a rapidly deteriorating emergency patient emphasize specific roles and assertive leadership (Wright et al., 2009), whereas skills that foster a learning and no-blame culture will emphasize flattened hierarchy, trust, collaborative conflict management, and individuals who flexibly move between different roles (Yeh et al., 2006; Moonaisur and Parumasur, 2012).

To make an effective contribution to a team, the new veterinarian will therefore need to understand their role and take responsibility for their actions, which will vary depending on the task and situation (Viner, 2010). Common elements of effective teams include trust and open communication (Moonaisur and Parumasur, 2012), and it is recommended that new graduate veterinarians take the opportunity to confirm their expected role in the team when they first start employment, particularly if their "team mates" are not what they are used to from veterinary school (e.g. the other veterinarians are located in a different practice site or work different shifts, the veterinary nurses, receptionists, and animal care colleagues that they work with). As a new graduate, it is important to take the opportunity to "learn the ropes" from the nursing team in the practice and to look for ways to contribute to workplace activities undertaken by employees at all levels. Taking this initiative will develop both collegial relationships and transferable skills that will help the new graduate in their current and future workplace roles.

Reflective Practice and Lifelong Learning

For the reflective professional, the first step of self-directed, reflective learning is identifying the desired outcome: the knowledge, skills, attributes, attitudes, and capacities that the veterinarian wishes to build and demonstrate. While students are frequently tempted to focus primarily on their clinical skills development (Matthew, et al., 2010; Matthew, et al., 2012), there are other competencies that are also critically important toward becoming a successful practitioner.

The next step is to compare this future "ideal self" with the reality of the "current self" (Goleman et al., 2002). The aim of this is to identify one's strengths (the areas where ideal and current selves overlap) and gaps (where ideal and current selves differ). It is then possible to create a "learning agenda" that allows the enhancing of strengths alongside the reduction of gaps. For example, workplace learning might provide the opportunity to engage with the more holistic elements of being a veterinarian, such as learning to take professional responsibility for the veterinarian–client collaboration in shared decision-making. Other useful areas of reflective focus might include developing an understanding of veterinary practice from across the different perspectives involved or learning better time management skills to balance one's professional and personal responsibilities (i.e. developing a balance between altruism and responsibility to patient and client vs. responsibility to one's self and personal health) (Matthew et al., 2012). If the workplace environment provides this range of learning opportunities, how might the veterinarian or student take advantage of them to enhance their personal development?

A learning agenda with goals that are specific, measurable, action-oriented, realistic, and time-limited (SMART) will help to focus reflection and feedback on performance and can be shared with a mentor (Jevring-Bäck and Bäck, 2007). Experimenting with new behaviors, thoughts and feelings, and practicing skills until mastery is established will enable progression toward one's goals (Goleman et al., 2002; Ericsson, 2004). Progressive development is facilitated by trusting relationships with mentors, colleagues, and others who support and encourage each step of this process.

Once performance goals have been set and progress toward them has started, specific events can be used to critically reflect on progress, adjusting actions, and/or goals as needed.

The process of critical reflection involves three stages that are outlined in Figure 9.1 (Boud et al., 1985; Freedman, 2007). First, the experience that one wishes to reflect upon is mentally revisited in order to recall and write down the specific events that occurred. Second, feelings encountered during the event are acknowledged to identify the personal impact and meaning of the situation. Third and finally, the experience is reevaluated by comparing one's personal performance at the time against the goals set, linking what was learned through the experience and any feedback obtained from others, with what was known beforehand. The final step of the critical reflection exercise is being committed to implementing a new action plan the next time a similar scenario arises. An important consideration of reflective learning is understanding that it is an ongoing process, targeted at improving one's personal management of increasingly complicated and challenging situations. Following a cycle of reflective learning, a subsequent difficult experience should not be seen as competence failure but should instead be viewed as a challenging opportunity for further reflection that will allow for setting of higher-reaching goals for next time.

The VetSet2Go website (www.vetset2go.edu.au) provides a useful online tool that can aid reflection and help self-assess effectiveness within the domains of task competence, employability, and adherence to professional values. This reflective self-assessment can be used to generate areas of focus for development (e.g. prior to a veterinary student's work placement or as part of appraisal or to enhance learning from an upcoming continuing education opportunity). More generally, it can be used as a reflective tool, analyzing confidence and/or performance within these domains in the context of a challenging situation experienced in practice (see Box 9.2).

Professional Identity Development

Professional identity – what is personally important and how personal goals for being a successful veterinarian are defined – develops constantly throughout one's career through repeated cycles of knowledge acquisition, experience, and reflection (Boud et al., 1985; Cruess and Cruess, 2006; Cruess et al., 2014). Identity is formed initially from family values and early childhood (Erikson, 1994). Wider social interactions, such as with friendship groups, and then through education and role models, continue to shape priorities and values, as individuals adhere firmly to some earlier beliefs and evolve their way of thinking about others (Erikson, 1994). Entering the veterinary workplace, initially during clinical rotations and then as a new graduate, represent critical moments in professional identity development, bringing exposure to

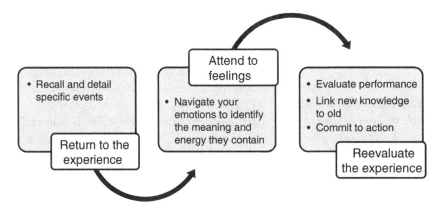

Figure 9.1 The critical reflection process.

Box 9.2   Example: Developing Clinical Consultation Skills Through Reflective Practice

A veterinary student undertaking clinic-based learning identifies that she would like to improve her clinical communication skills and wants to address each element of an effective consultation individually. She asks her supervisor, Dr. Smith, whether she would be willing to provide feedback on how well the client consultation is initiated. Dr. Smith agrees.

The student shares two SMART goals that she would like to work on with Dr. Smith:

1) *To greet the client and patient by name before inviting them into the consultation room*
2) *To introduce myself and my role at the start of the interaction*

The consultation in the reception area is soon initiated by the student greeting the client by name and introducing herself and her role. The student is taken aback when the client exclaims "You're late!" picks up their pet and brushes past the student into the consultation room before she has the chance to greet the patient as well. She follows the client into the consultation room, only to find the client glaring at her and tapping their foot impatiently. The student says quickly "Dr. Smith will be consulting with you today" and then steps back and falls silent while her supervisor takes over the consultation. As Dr. Smith talks to the client, the student mulls over how rude the client was to interrupt her greeting and push past into the consultation room.

After the consultation concludes, the student and Dr. Smith debrief. The student acknowledges that, while she completed her first SMART goal successfully, she only partially completed her second goal. "It was the client's fault!" she exclaims. "They never gave me a chance. They were so rude!" It is clear that she is still feeling angry.

Dr. Smith agrees with the student's assessment of her performance against her goals and then asks whether she might be open to additional feedback on her performance. Warily, the student agrees. Dr. Smith then invites the student to reflect on why she is feeling so angry about the way the client acted. After reflection, the student realizes that courtesy and respect are behaviors she greatly values. The client behaved in a way that violated these values, and this caused the student's initial surprise and subsequent anger. Dr. Smith then asks about the impact of the client's reaction on the student's performance. After thinking back to the consultation, the student acknowledges that her surprise at how the client acted made her miss any opportunity to apologize for being late before greeting the pet as planned, and then her subsequent anger distracted her from focusing on observing what Dr. Smith did to build the relationship with the client after the challenging start to the consultation.

The student decides that the next time a client behaves in a rude manner, she will pause before entering the consultation room to take a deep breath and privately acknowledge her feelings. Dr. Smith extended her critical reflection on the student's performance with a reminder to always consider the client's perspective and to avoid taking the client's behavior personally. Together these actions will help the student to refocus on the goal of successfully initiating the consultation.

---

values and views of the veterinary role that might be different to those encountered previously. The reflective professional draws on these critical experiences (such as incidences of conflict or uncertainty, or observation of positive role models) and considers them in light of their relevant developing knowledge base. Decisions are then made about which personal beliefs are non-negotiable and which might be more amenable to development. Identity is then adapted and reconsidered in light of new experiences and social interactions.

Identity is important because of the feelings evoked when the veterinarian acts in a way that aligns with (i.e. affording a sense of positivity) or is discordant with (i.e. evoking a sense of frustration and distress) their professional values, and provides a sense of career success and satisfaction based on being able to achieve personal veterinary goals. There will inevitably be occasions when a veterinarian's decisions directly conflict with their ideal veterinary self (i.e. the veterinarian they aspire to be). These situations may prove stressful and personally disappointing. Resilience will, in part, depend on the manner on the context of the situation: do these difficult situations represent a temporary, conscious compromise from one's professional identity, because empathizing with and supporting others is also valued? Alternatively, are the actions taken in a situation perceived as chronic and long-term examples of behavior that runs counter to the desired identity of the veterinarian, resulting in ongoing frustrations with achieving professional goals? In the latter case, when the veterinarian feels chronically frustrated at not being able to make decisions that align with their professional identity, it becomes important for them to reflect on their personal goals, and consider whether or not colleagues and peers could have achieved these goals in a similar work environment. If they believe that their colleagues would have been more effective in enacting their professional goals in a specific situation, then it is a good idea to talk to them. Using role models to help identify personal competence gaps enables the veterinarian to take future actions that align with their professional goals. It can be very challenging when prioritized personal beliefs appear misaligned with the apparent expected behaviors of the workplace, and this leads to reflection regarding one's values, and whether they should be adapted. When reflection determines that one's values are of utmost importance and cannot be compromised, it will be necessary to find ways to integrate these values in one's professional actions. This might require the learning of additional competencies (such as communication skills or conflict management) or even the researching of alternative professional environments, where the workplace norms better align with their personal values.

Conclusion

This chapter has reviewed some of the core skills that are required for effective veterinary clinical practice besides those performed hands-on. Decision-making in situations of complexity and uncertainty, such as in the example of the sick puppy given at the start of the chapter, requires effective communication, collaboration, and conflict resolution skills that are underpinned by emotional intelligence. Lifelong learning, teamwork, and reflective practice enable the veterinarian to build their capacity for resilience to practice stressors and help the practitioner achieve long-term career fulfillment. Reflecting on one's professional identity influences the meaning of individual and team success in practice. The successful veterinarian focuses not only on their technical abilities but also works to achieve growth in these other important areas of competence as well.

References

Adams, C. L., Frankel, R. M. 2007. It may be a dog's life but the relationship with her owners is also key to her health and well being: communication in veterinary medicine. *Vet Clin North Am Small Anim Pract*, 37, 1–17.

Adams C. L., Kurtz, S. 2017. *Skills for Communicating in Veterinary Medicine*. Oxford, UK: Otmoor Publishing.

Arbe Montoya A. I., Hazel, S., Matthew, S. M., et al. 2019. Moral distress in veterinarians. *Vet Rec*, 185, 631.

Armitage-Chan, E., Maddison, J., May, S. A. 2016. What is the veterinary professional identity? Preliminary findings from web-based continuing professional development in veterinary professionalism. *Vet Rec*, 178, 318.

Armitage-Chan, E., May, S. A. 2018. Identity, environment and mental wellbeing in the veterinary profession. *Vet Rec*, 183, 68.

Armitage-Chan, E. 2019a, 'I wish I was someone else': Complexities in identity formation and professional wellbeing in veterinary surgeons. *Vet Rec*, 187, 113.

Armitage-Chan, E., 2019b. Best practice in supporting professional identity formation: Use of a professional reasoning framework. *J Vet Med Educ*, 47, 125–136.

Batchelor, C. E. M., McKeegan, D. E. F. 2012. Survey of the frequency and perceived stressfulness of ethical dilemmas encountered in UK veterinary practice. *Vet Rec*, 170, 19.

Boud, D., Keogh, R., Walker, D. 1985, Promoting reflection in learning: A model. In: *Reflection: Turning Experience into Learning*. Boud, D., Keogh, R., Walker, D. (eds.) Kogan Page, London.

Cake, M. A., Bell, M. A., Bickley, N., et al. 2015. The life of meaning: A model of the positive contributions to well-being from veterinary work. *J Vet Med Educ*, 42, 184–193.

Cake, M. A., McArthur, M., Matthew, S. M., et al. 2017. Finding the balance: Uncovering resilience in the veterinary literature. *J Vet Med Educ*, 44, 95–105.

Cake, M., McArthur, M. L., Mansfield, C. F., et al. 2019. Challenging identity: Development of a measure of veterinary career motivations. *Vet Rec*, 186, 386.

Carver, C. S. 1997. You want to measure coping but your protocol's too long: Consider the brief COPE. *Int J Behav Med*, 4, 92–100.

Cerney, M. S., Buskirk, J. R. 1991. Anger: The hidden part of grief. *Bull Menninger Clin*, 55, 228–237.

Clarke, C. A., Knights, D. 2018. Practice makes perfect? Skillful performances in veterinary work. *Hum Relat*, 71, 1395–1421.

Coe, J. B., Adams, C. L., Bonnett, B. N. 2007. A focus group study of veterinarians' and pet owners' perceptions of the monetary aspects of veterinary care. *J Am Vet Med Assoc*, 231, 1510–1518.

Coe, J. B., Adams, C. L., Bonnett, B. N. 2009. Prevalence and nature of cost discussions during clinical appointments in companion animal practice. *J Am Vet Med Assoc*, 234, 1418–1424.

Cornell, K. K., Kopcha, M. 2007, Client-veterinarian communication: Skills for client centered dialogue and shared decision making. *Vet Clin North Am Small Anim Pract*, 37, 37–47.

Cruess, R. L., Cruess, S. R. 2006. Teaching professionalism: General principles. *Med Teach*, 28, 205–208.

Cruess, R. L., Cruess, S. R., Boudreau, J. D., et al. 2014. Reframing medical education to support professional identity formation. *Acad Med*, 89, 1446–1451.

Demerouti, E., Bakker, A. B., Nachreiner, F., et al. 2001. The job demands-resources model of burnout. *J Appl Psychol*, 86, 499–512.

Ericsson, K. A. 2004. Deliberate practice and the acquisition and maintenance of expert performance in medicine and related domains. *Acad Med*, 79, S70–S81.

Erikson, E. H. 1994. *Identity and the Life Cycle*. New York, USA: WW Norton & Company.

Freedman, J. 2007. *At the Heart of Leadership: How to Get Results with Emotional Intelligence*. San Mateo, CA: Six Seconds.

Gardner, D. H., Hini, D. 2006. Work-related stress in the veterinary profession in New Zealand. *N Z Vet J*, 54, 119–124.

Goleman, D. 1998. *Working with Emotional Intelligence*. London, UK: Bloomsbury.

Goleman, D., Boyatzis, R., McKee, A. 2002. *Primal Leadership: Realizing the Power of Emotional Intelligence*, Boston, USA: Harvard Business School Press.

Gregório, H., Santos, P., Pires, I., et al. 2016. Comparison of veterinary health services expectations and perceptions between oncologic pet owners, non-oncologic pet owners and veterinary staff using the SERVQUAL methodology. *Vet World*, 9, 1275–1281.

Grimm, H., Bergadano, A., Musk, G. C., et al. 2018. Drawing the line in clinical treatment of companion animals: recommendations from an ethics working party. *Vet Rec*, 182, 664.

Halpern, J. 2007. Empathy and patient–physician conflicts. *J Gen Intern Med*, 22, 696–700.

Hughes, K., Rhind, S. M., Mossop, L., et al. 2018. 'Care about my animal, know your stuff and take me seriously': United Kingdom and Australian clients' views on the capabilities most important in their veterinarians. *Vet Rec*, 183, 534.

Jevring-Bäck, C., Bäck, E. 2007. *Managing a Veterinary Practice*, 2nd Edition. Elsevier Saunders: Edinburgh.

Kinnison, T., Guile, D., May, S. A. 2015. Errors in veterinary practice: Preliminary lessons for building better veterinary teams. *Vet Rec*, 177, 492.

Kipperman, B. S., Kass, P. H., Rishniw, M. 2017. Factors that influence small animal veterinarians' opinions and actions regarding cost of care and effects of economic limitations on patient care and outcome and professional career satisfaction and burnout. *J Am Vet Med Assoc*, 250, 785–794.

Koole, S. L., Jostmann, N. B. 2004. Getting a grip on your feelings: Effects of action orientation and external demands on intuitive affect regulation. *J Pers Soc Psychol*, 87, 974–990.

Lencioni, P. 2008. *The Five Dysfunctions of a Team: An Illustrated Leadership Fable.* Singapore: John Wiley & Sons.

Mansfield, C. F., Beltman, S., Broadley, T., et al. 2016. Building resilience in teacher education: An evidenced informed framework. *Teach Teach Educ*, 54, 77–87.

Mastenbroek, N. J. J. M. 2017. The art of staying engaged: The role of personal resources in the mental well-being of young veterinary professionals. *J Vet Med Educ*, 44, 84–94.

Mastenbroek, N. J. J. M., Jaarsma, A. D. C., Demerouti, E., et al. 2014. Burnout and engagement, and its predictors in young veterinary professionals: The influence of gender. *Vet Rec*, 174, 144.

Matthew, S. M., Taylor, R. M., Ellis, R. A. 2010. Students' experiences of clinic-based learning during a final year veterinary internship programme. *High Educ Res & Dev*, 29, 389–404.

Matthew, S. M., Taylor, R. M., Ellis, R. A. 2012. Relationships between students' experiences of learning in an undergraduate internship programme and new graduates' experiences of professional practice. *High Educ*, 64, 529–542.

Mayer, J. D., Salovey, P. 1997. What is emotional intelligence? In: *Emotional Development and Emotional Intelligence: Educational Implications.* Salovey, P. Sluyter, D. (eds.) New York: Basic Books, pp. 3–31.

McArthur, M., Mansfield, C., Matthew, S., et al. 2017. Resilience in veterinary students and the predictive role of mindfulness and self-compassion. *J Vet Med Educ*, 44, 106–115.

McArthur, M. L., Matthew, S. M., Brand, C. P. B., et al. 2019. Cross-sectional analysis of veterinary student coping strategies and stigma in seeking psychological help. *Vet Rec*, 184, 709.

Moonaisur, D., Parumasur, S. B. 2012. Perceived enablers and obstacles to team effectiveness. *Corp Ownersh Control*, 10, 521–534.

Moore, I. C., Coe, J. B., Adams, C. L., et al. 2014. The role of veterinary team effectiveness in job satisfaction and burnout in companion animal veterinary clinics. *J Am Vet Med Assoc*, 245, 513–524.

Moses, L., Malowney, M. J., Wesley Boyd, J. 2018. Ethical conflict and moral distress in veterinary practice: A survey of North American veterinarians. *J Vet Intern Med*, 32, 2115–2122.

Mullan, S., Main, D. 2001. Ethical decision-making in veterinary practice. *Vet Rec*, 149, 339.

Philip, J., Gold, M., Schwarz, M., et al. 2007. Anger in palliative care: a clinical approach. *Intern Med J*, 37, 49–55.

Platt, B., Hawton, K., Simkin, S., et al. 2012. Suicidal behaviour and psychosocial problems in veterinary surgeons: A systematic review. *Soc Psychiatry Psyciatr Epidemiol*, 47, 223–240.

RCVS. 2018. Code of Professional Conduct for Veterinary Surgeons. https://www.rcvs.org.uk/setting-standards/advice-and-guidance/code-of-professional-conduct-for-veterinary-surgeons/ Accessed February 15, 2021.

Robertson, K. 2005. Active listening: More than just paying attention. *Aust Fam Physician*, 34, 1053–1055.

Ruby, K. L., DeBowes, R. M. 2007, The veterinary health care team: Going from good to great. *Vet Clin North Am Small Anima Pract*, 37, 19–35.

Ryan, R. M., Deci, E. L. 2000. Self-determination theory and the facilitation of intrinsic motivation, social development, and well-being. *Am Psychol*, 55, 68–78.

Seligman, M. E. P. 2006. *Learned Optimism: How to Change Your Mind and Your Life*. New York: Vintage Books.

Shaw, J. R. 2006. Four core communication skills of highly effective practitioners. *Vet Clin North Am Small Anima Pract*, 36, 385–396.

Silverman, J., Kurtz, S., Draper, J. 2005. *Skills for Communicating with Patients*, 2nd Edition. Abingdon, UK: Radcliffe Publishing Ltd.

Thomas, K. W. 1992. Conflict and conflict management: Reflections and update. *J Organ Behav*, 13, 265–274.

Tomlin, J. L., Brodbelt, D. C., May, S. A. 2010. Influences on the decision to study veterinary medicine: Variation with sex and background. *Vet Rec*, 166, 744.

Viner, B. 2010. *Success in Veterinary Practice: Maximising Clinical Outcomes and Personal Well-Being*. Chichester, UK: Wiley-Blackwell.

Volk, J. O., Felsted, K. E., Thomas, J. G., et al. 2011. Executive summary of the bayer veterinary care usage study. *J Am Vet Med Assoc*, 238, 1275–1282.

Wright, M. C., Phillips-Bute, B. G., Petrusa, E. R., et al. 2009. Assessing teamwork in medical education and practice: relating behavioural teamwork ratings and clinical performance. *Med Teach*, 31, 30–38.

Yeh, E., Smith, C., Jennings, C., et al. 2006. Team building: A 3-dimensional teamwork model. *Team Perform Manag*, 12, 192–197.

Appendix 1

OSCEs (Objective Structured Clinical Examinations)

The following OSCE examples are provided by clinical skills teams for the purposes of sharing how these examinations are conducted in various different institutions. The examples presented include grading rubrics with binary checklists (yes or no; 1 or 0), as well as a GRS (global rating scale).

Elements of OSCEs included in some of the examples in this appendix:

Scene, Student task, Student information – This portion of the OSCE text is posted for students to read as they enter the station (The Ohio State University OSCEs).

Critical error – Student commits a grave safety mistake that might hurt the patient, hurt the student, or hurt the examiner. The examiner stops the exam and the student has to repeat the station at a later date after feedback and further practice.

Mandatory station failure – Example OSCE # 9 includes an example of listing reasons why a student would automatically fail the station despite their actual accumulated score.

Stop and restart – If a student makes a minor mistake that is unacceptable during the skill or procedure but it is not considered a "grave safety mistake," then the examiner may stop the student and start them again at an earlier time point in the examination. This penalizes the student for making the mistake by reducing the time they have to complete the station, but avoids them having to repeat the entire station.

Feedback from examiner – Each examiner is asked to complete the feedback form to allow for future improvements to the station and to collect feedback regarding performance of the student cohort that can be shared with the class as a whole for generic feedback immediately after the exam. This class feedback lessens class anxiety while they are waiting for their individual results and helps reinforce a growth mindset by reminding students that everyone has items to work upon.

1) Making a cheese and pickle sandwich – Sarah Baillie and Rachel Harris, University of Bristol, and Emma Read, The Ohio State University. This OSCE is used for training students to help familiarize them with the exam procedure and is also useful for training examiners. Other similar examples include "making a peanut butter and jelly sandwich" (University of Calgary) or "making a cup of tea" (University of Bristol).

2) Gowning and gloving (GRS checklist) – Tatiana Motta and Emma Read, The Ohio State University. This OSCE includes a GRS checklist where individual steps in the procedure are lumped together into broader categories that are scored on a Likert scale with anchors. This prevents rater fatigue

Veterinary Clinical Skills, First Edition. Edited by Emma K. Read, Matt R. Read, and Sarah Baillie.
© 2022 John Wiley & Sons, Inc. Published 2022 by John Wiley & Sons, Inc.
Companion website: www.wiley.com/go/read/veterinary

with long checklists and also helps to better discriminate between more advanced learners by focusing on finer details.

3) Draping a small animal patient for abdominal surgery – Tatiana Motta, The Ohio State University. This OSCE includes the "stop and restart" method of managing student error. Figures are included to clarify the finer details of drape handling to examiners.

4) Bovine surgical anatomy – Jennifer Schleining, Texas A & M University. This OSCE is an example of how knowledge components might be tested as part of the exam.

5) Canine physical exam – Steven Horvath and Missy Matusicky, The Ohio State University. This physical exam station includes some useful items for assessing physical exam skills no matter what the species. The rectal temperature information is provided in advance so that students do not need to perform this (better for the patient!). A double binaural stethoscope is used to make sure that the student is able to auscultate the chest and accurately determine the heart rate. This OSCE is not only testing what the student "does" but also asks them to verbalize information to the examiner. Note that this is made clear to the student in the "student task" section. This OSCE includes a critical error related to patient safety.

6) Surgical towel placement – Abi Taylor, North Carolina State University. This simple OSCE checklist includes the student information briefly at the top.

7) Pedicle ligature (two-handed tie) – Abi Taylor, North Carolina State University. This simple OSCE checklist includes the student information briefly at the top.

8) Equine handling and restraint – Teresa Burns and Emma Read, The Ohio State University. This OSCE includes a critical error related to patient safety. Note that the checklist includes differential points for various items with those related to safety and the central aspect of the task being weighted most heavily.

9) Intramuscular injection in a canine model – Julie Williamson, Lincoln Memorial University. This OSCE includes a list of reasons why a student would automatically fail the station despite their score (mandatory station failure).

10) Anesthetic machine set up and leak testing – Matt Read, MedVet, and Carolina Ricco Pereira, The Ohio State University. This OSCE is an example of a critical skill related to patient safety. Students rarely if ever argue that an OSCE such as this is a fair test of their knowledge and skill!

Making a Cheese and Pickle Sandwich

Sarah Baillie[1], Rachel Harris[1], and Emma K. Read[2]

[1]*Bristol Veterinary School, University of Bristol, Bristol, United Kingdom*
[2]*College of Veterinary Medicine, The Ohio State University, Columbus, OH, USA*

	Examiner Initials:	**OSCE Station: Making a Cheese and Pickle Sandwich**
	Date:	*Mail merge:*
Instructions for examiners: • Ask '***Your name is. . .?***' • Check this against the details on the right. • Then ask: '***Have you read the scenario?***' • Then ask '***Do you understand what you have to do?***' Then say: '***Please begin.***'		*OSCE GROUP* *STUDENT NAME* *CANDIDATE NUMBER*

	Insert a score of '1' if the candidate demonstrates the item, and '0' if they do not:	**'1' or '0'**
1	Starts by putting on gloves	
2	Selects two slices of bread	
3	Place bread on paper plate	
4	Selects butter knife	
5	Spreads butter/equivalent on one side of each slice of bread	
6	Selects kitchen knife	
7	Cuts pieces of cheese	
8	Use chopping board to cut cheese on	
9	Puts cheese onto one slice of bread	
10	Uses separate butter knife for pickle	
11	Spreads pickle on cheese or other slice of bread	
12	Does not "double dip" into pickle jar after contact with sandwich	
13	Places two pieces of bread together to make sandwich	
14	Cuts sandwich in half	
15	Observes food safety protocols throughout	
16	Handles knives safely	
Total Achieved (examiner please add up total score):		**/16**

Global Rating Scale (☑):	☐ Bad Fail	☐ Just Fail	☐ Just Pass	☐ Good Pass

Comments (*e.g. reason for fail, any incidents that occurred*):

Veterinary Clinical Skills, First Edition. Edited by Emma K. Read, Matt R. Read, and Sarah Baillie.
© 2022 John Wiley & Sons, Inc. Published 2022 by John Wiley & Sons, Inc.
Companion website: www.wiley.com/go/read/veterinary

Notes

- This OSCE is used as a demonstration to prepare students for the OSCE process (i.e. OSCE etiquette, sound system, do's and don'ts, etc.), allowing them to then concentrate on practising the skill or procedure. It is also used in examiner training.
- The demonstration is usually run as a 'play' at the front of a lecture theatre. Allow plenty of time for questions.

- The original OSCE was a 'Peanut Butter & Jam Sandwich' developed at the University of Calgary, Canada by Emma Read and Darlene Donszelmann. It has been adapted with permission by University of Bristol, UK.
- A YouTube video of this OSCE is available at: https://youtu.be/5mP4Jmxf9mc

Authors: Sarah Baillie & Rachel Harris, University of Bristol, UK; Emma Read, The Ohio State University, USA and Darlene Donszelmann, University of Calgary

Asepsis – Gowning and Closed Gloving

Tatiana Motta and Emma K. Read

College of Veterinary Medicine, The Ohio State University, Columbus, OH, USA

<u>Learning Outcomes - This station will test the candidate's ability to:</u>

- Select and organize the supplies needed for the task.
- Respect principles of asepsis by showing awareness of themselves and their surroundings.
- Perform with dexterity while drying hands, gowning, and closed gloving.
- Work in a smooth, efficient, and precise manner.
- Achieve an adequate final product: surgeon ready to operate.

Case Scenario and Candidate Tasks

<u>Scene:</u>

You are performing your first surgery today. You have just completed an aseptic hand scrub and will now need to <u>gown and closed glove</u>.

<u>Candidate Task:</u>

1 Set up and prepare for gowning and closed gloving.
2 There is no need to scrub your hands (pretend this has been done already) – start with drying your hands instead.
3 Put on your sterile surgical gown.
4 Put on your sterile gloves using closed gloving technique.
5 Respect the principles of aseptic technique at all times.
6 The examiner may help you, if required, but you must tell them exactly what you need.
7 Your examiner may ask you to **"stop and restart"** if you commit a breach in aseptic technique that you do not recognize.

Veterinary Clinical Skills, First Edition. Edited by Emma K. Read, Matt R. Read, and Sarah Baillie.
© 2022 John Wiley & Sons, Inc. Published 2022 by John Wiley & Sons, Inc.
Companion website: www.wiley.com/go/read/veterinary

Examiner's Information

Examiner's Information:

1 Select and organize the supplies needed for the task: student should put on a cap first, and a mask second. The mask should be firmly tightened with the top tie tied at the crown of the head and the second (lower) tie tied at the nape of the neck (both on the outside of the cap). The colored side of the mask should be facing out (so it is visible to the examiner). All hair should be within the cap.

2 The candidate should:
   - Respect principles of asepsis and show awareness of themselves and their surroundings.
   - Show dexterity while drying hands, as well as when gowning and closed gloving.
   - Work in a smooth, efficient, and precise manner.
   - Achieve an adequate final product: A surgeon ready to operate.

3 If the candidate fails to start the appropriate task, then the examiner should state, **"Would you like to please re-read the scenario?"**

4 If the candidate commits a breach in aseptic technique and does not correct it or mention this to you within the next 5–10 seconds, please tell the student to **"stop and restart"** from the point of contamination (examiner should use discretion in how far back to "rewind" the student). As an example, a student might touch their mask with a gloved hand. If the student does not say anything within the next 5–10 seconds, ask the student to stop, and restart at closed gloving. The examiner will need to remove the contaminated gloves from the student's hands and then will open a new set of gloves for the student to put on.

At the end of the task, the examiner needs to:

Clean up the station: remove and discard used disposable supplies.

Place a new wrapped gown on the table.

Place the used gowns and gloves into the bins provided for recycling.

Grading for Gowning and Gloving

Please circle the numbers below that best describe the candidate's ability to do the following:

Global Rating Score Choose only one per dimension (1–5)	Clearly below expectations		Acceptable performance		Performs above expectations
1 **Organization and material selection**	1	2	3	4	5
	Stops to think and readjust multiple times. Forgets to wear cap/mask. Starts performance without having materials ready		Occasionally stops to think or readjusts motions to maintain organization. Starts performance and has to ask for some materials because not thoroughly prepared		Effective and confident motions. All materials are ready before performance starts. Rings/watch are removed. Needs no extra help to perform task

2 **Dexterity while gowning**	1	2	3	4	5
	Major deficiencies on performance. Lacks dexterity during multiple steps		Able to perform skill and able to deal with breaches of sterility. Tentative hand motions or movements but able to complete task		Effective and confident in every step involved: drying hands, picking up gown, unfolding it and inserting hands into the sleeves. Excellent dexterity
3 **Dexterity while gloving**	1	2	3	4	5
	Major deficiencies in performance. Lacks dexterity during multiple steps		Able to perform skill and able to deal with breaches of sterility. Tentative hand motions or movements but able to complete task		Effective, precise and confident in every step involved: opening the wrappers, grasping the gloves while fingers are still in the cuff, adjusting each fingers and cuffs at the end. Excellent dexterity
4 **Recognition regarding sterility**	1	2	3	4	5
	Commits breaches of sterility with no recognition		Occasionally commits minor errors in asepsis that are recognized and corrected		Always conscious of surroundings. Superior attention to asepsis. Demonstrates understanding of sterile vs. clean technique
5 **Quality of final product**	1	2	3	4	5
	Inferior performance. Surgical attire improperly fitted or applied		Acceptably attired with room for some improvement in placement or fit of cap, mask, gown and gloves		Perfectly applied surgical attire including fit and placement of all components

Critical errors:

None

Number of attempts taken to gown:_____
Re-wind needed to gown? ☐ no ☐ yes, once ☐ yes, more than once
Number of attempts taken to closed gloving:_____
Re-wind needed to closed glove? ☐ no ☐ yes, once ☐ yes, more than once
Complete with time to spare: ☐ 1 minute or less, ☐ 1-2 minutes, ☐ 2-3 minutes, ☐ more than 3 minutes.

Global rating scale performance (*this will be used to calculate the passing/failing grade*):

Unable to Perform	Borderline	Satisfactory	Very Good	Excellent

Open comments:

Station Equipment and Materials

State the required equipment for 1 station. The OSCE will have 5 to 15 stations total:			
Item	**Amount**	**Brand**	**Specific Comments**
Sterile gloves	Many		(in various sizes – from 6 to 8 1/2)
Sterile nitrile gloves	Many		for those with allergies, variable sizes
Sterile gowns in various sizes	Many		S-XXL
Caps	30		
Masks	30		
Normal garbage can	1		
Container to collect used gowns	1		

State the required equipment to reset this station between candidates			
Item	**Amount**	**Brand**	**Specific Comments**
none			

Feedback from examiner:

Please share your opinion and experience so we can improve this station for next year:

1. What worked well for this station?

   _____
   _____
   _____

2. Opportunities for improvement of this station:

   _____
   _____
   _____

3. Any additional information regarding pros and cons of each:

   a) Simulator_____
   b) Checklist/packet_____
   c) Supplies_____
   d) Time_____

Info to be shared with the students during the debriefing video created after the end of the exams:

1. Top 3 most proficient steps observed:

   _____
   _____
   _____

2. Top 3 most deficient steps observed:

   _____
   _____
   _____

Examiner's last name: _____ Thanks for helping us today!!

Asepsis – Draping

Tatiana Motta

College of Veterinary Medicine, The Ohio State University, Columbus, OH, USA

Learning Outcomes - This station will test the student's ability to:
1 Apply principles of asepsis. 2 Drape a patient in preparation for an abdominal procedure.

Scene:
Your patient has been aseptically prepared and is in now ready to be draped for an abdominal procedure.

Case Scenario and Candidate Tasks

Student Task:
You are to: 1 Use the materials provided to drape the simulated patient. 2 Use a two-layer draping technique. 3 Secure drapes to the patient. 4 Follow principles of asepsis at all times. 5 The examiner may help you, if required, but you must tell the examiner exactly what they have to do. 6 Your examiner may ask you to **"stop and restart"** if you commit a breach in aseptic technique while draping. You will be able to restart; however, your time will not restart and you will have the time remaining on the clock. You will NOT need to re-gown or re-glove.

Veterinary Clinical Skills, First Edition. Edited by Emma K. Read, Matt R. Read, and Sarah Baillie.
© 2022 John Wiley & Sons, Inc. Published 2022 by John Wiley & Sons, Inc.
Companion website: www.wiley.com/go/read/veterinary

Examiner's Information

Examiner's Information:

1 Students should arrive at the station wearing: surgical cap, mask, surgical gown, and sterile gloves. The simulated patient has already been prepped for them and is ready to be draped.

2 A two-layer draping technique must be used. The first layer is composed of four field drapes (four-corner drapes) that should be placed with the edge folded forward (toward the patient). Students must hold the smaller drapes using the correct technique to avoid contamination of gloved fingers (see image of that below).

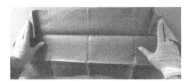

3 Drapes must be secured to the patient using towel clamps (taking substantial bite of the simulated model, not just the fur). Students may apply a lot of force while using towel clamps because these simulated patients are extremely soft – this is acceptable in this model situation. Placing towel clamps backwards (so the handles are extending into the draped field) is not acceptable and should be corrected by the student before the top drape (oversheet) is placed. Feel free to ask the student to demonstrate that the towel clamps are engaged into the simulated skin – they should respond by giving them a firm tug, which allows you to see how well they are properly anchored.

4 Top drapes (oversheet) can be placed by the student alone or examiner help may be requested.

5 Principles of asepsis must be followed at all times. Common breaches of asepsis that occur: student's gown touches the patient or the table while applying the quarter (smaller) drapes. Student itch their mask with gloved hands. Finger of student touches unprepped areas of the patient. Student places drape and towel clamps before deciding to move it and then reclamps, penetrating drape a second time.

6 The examiner may help the student, if required, but the student must describe exactly what the examiner should do. If asking for examiner's help, student must describe that only the inside (lighter color) of the drape can be touched by the non-sterile helper.

7 If a student contaminates themselves but recognizes it and verbalizes it to you within 5–10 seconds, the student should not lose points for that line item in the checklist. If a student contaminates themselves and proceed for longer than 5–10 seconds without recognizing it, then the examiner should say "**Please stop and restart.**" The examiner determines from where they want the student to begin again. Students will not re-gown or re-glove (because of the length of time involved) but will lose points for that item in the checklist and the clock will not stop – they have the time remaining on the clock.

8 If the student fails to start the appropriate task or gets off task, then the examiner should state, "**Would you like to please re-read the scenario?**" For example, a student may start placing the top drape before the four corner drapes are placed, or use perforation clamps on the top drape. The examiner must wait 5–10 seconds before stating the sentence above to give the student the opportunity to fix it themselves.

At the end of the task, the examiner needs to:

1 Undrape the simulator.

2 Replace drapes if torn.

3 Place surgical instruments back onto the table in same position.

Draping Station Checklist/Grading

The student should do the following:	<u>Yes</u>	<u>No</u>	Points
1 Each field drape held at correct height – no higher than shoulders, and no lower than waist.			1
2 No contamination for field drapes: Surgeon bends at the waist, their gown never touches undraped table.			2
3 No contamination for field drapes: Surgeon's gloves are fully protected by the field drape being turned back at corners.			2
4 The fold of the drape faces forward (toward the patient), not backwards (toward the surgeon) for each drape.			1
5 The first two drapes are placed at the cranial and caudal aspects of the patient (and are not placed as lateral drapes).			1
6 All 4 field drapes on surgical field are placed correctly – dragged from center back to periphery, but never pushed up from periphery toward center.			1
7 Correct tripod grip handling of all towel clamps.			1
8 Penetrating towel clamps are placed correctly (backwards towel clamps with handles extending into the central field must be called out by the examiner if the student does not correct it within 5–10 seconds)			1
9 Ensures the skin is engaged by each of the four towel clamps. Examiners says: "Please raise each of the towel clamps to show me that the skin is engaged"			1
10 Top drape (oversheet) is placed over the center of the patient/table like an "open book."			1
11 Starts unfolding the top drape only after the field drapes have been secured on the patient.			1
12 One hand keeps the top drape from moving around, while the other hand unfolds the drape.			1
13 While draping, student opens the drape successfully on own or asks for examiner's help.			1
14 No contamination for oversheet: Surgeon bends at the waist, their gown never touches undraped table.			2
15 No contamination for oversheet: Surgeon's gloves are fully protected by the drapes and kept above the waist, below the shoulders.			2
16 Top drape is secured in place with non-penetrating clamps.			2
	Total Points:		21

<u>**Critical Errors:**</u>

None

Global rating scale performance (*this will be used to calculate the passing/failing grades*):

Unable to Perform	Borderline	Satisfactory	Very Good	Excellent

Open comments from examiner to student:

Station Equipment and Materials

State the required equipment for this station:		
Item	Amount	Specific Comments
Simulated patient ready for draping	1/station	Ikea dog, 4 suction cups, 2 bungee cords and 1 skin simulator with grommets
Mayo stand	1/station	
Mayo stand covers	1/station	
Surgical towels	1/station	Used to cover the mayo stand
Field drapes	5/station	
Top drape – with pre-cut slit (rectangle)	2/station	The pre-cut slit must be at the center of the drape and match the size of the "prepped area" on the skin simulator
Towel clamps	8/station	
Mosquito hemostats	8/station	
Normal garbage can	1/station	
Step stool	1/station	For short students
Plastic tub container to store top drapes that need to be refolded	1/station	

Feedback from examiner:

Please share your opinion and experience so we can improve this station for next year:

1. What worked well for this station?

   _____
   _____
   _____
   _____

2. Opportunities for improvement of this station:

   _____
   _____
   _____

3. Any additional information regarding pros and cons of each:

   a) Simulator_____
   b) Checklist/packet _____
   c) Supplies_____
   d) Time _____

Info to be shared with the students during the debriefing video that will be made after the end of the exams:

1. Top 3 most proficient steps observed:

   _____
   _____
   _____

2. Top 3 most deficient steps observed:

   _____
   _____
   _____

THANKS for helping us today!!

Bovine Anatomy and Surgical Landmarks - Part One

Jennifer Schleining

COLLEGE OF VETERINARY MEDICINE & BIOMEDICAL SCIENCES

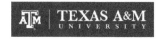

OSCE Station: Live Animal Station – Bovine Anatomy and Surgical Landmarks

<u>**Checklist**</u>   Dr. Jennifer Schleining

PLACE STUDENT ID STICKER HERE

	Student performed the following:	Yes (1)	No (0)
1	Demonstrated an awareness of safety around the animal, chute and gates		
2	Palpated for the transverse vertebral processes in the proximal paralumbar fossa caudal to the 13th rib		
3	Correctly identified L1, L2, or L4 according to the card drawn by placing a sticker on the correct transverse vertebral process		
4	Correctly identified the location of the dermatome supplied by the nerve blocked at their selected landmark		
5	Correctly identified the nerve that is blocked at their selected landmark on the exam sheet		
6	Identifies the block as the distal paravertebral nerve block, Cakala nerve block, or Cakala-Delahanty nerve block on the exam sheet		
	TOTAL CONTENT MARKS	/	

Veterinary Clinical Skills, First Edition. Edited by Emma K. Read, Matt R. Read, and Sarah Baillie.
© 2022 John Wiley & Sons, Inc. Published 2022 by John Wiley & Sons, Inc.
Companion website: www.wiley.com/go/read/veterinary

Bovine Anatomy and Surgical Landmarks - Part Two

Jennifer Schleining

**COLLEGE OF VETERINARY MEDICINE
& BIOMEDICAL SCIENCES**

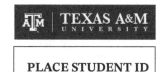

**OSCE Station: Bovine Anatomy and
Surgical Landmarks**   Dr. Jennifer Schleining

**PLACE STUDENT ID
STICKER HERE**

1. Identify and place a sticker at the location of the transverse vertebral process of the 1st lumbar vertebrae.

2. Record on the line below the name of the nerve that is blocked if lidocaine is injected at this site.

   _____

3. Record the name of the local block if lidocaine is deposited above and below the ventral vertebral process at your identified site.

   _____

4. Place one sticker in the center of the dermatome that is supplied by this nerve.

5. Hand this card to your station monitor.

   _____

**If you finish your station before time is complete, stand and wait quietly until you are
released by the room monitor.**

Veterinary Clinical Skills, First Edition. Edited by Emma K. Read, Matt R. Read, and Sarah Baillie.
© 2022 John Wiley & Sons, Inc. Published 2022 by John Wiley & Sons, Inc.
Companion website: www.wiley.com/go/read/veterinary

Canine Physical Exam

Steven Horvath and Missy Matusicky

College of Veterinary Medicine, The Ohio State University, Columbus, OH, USA

Learning Outcomes - This station will test the student's ability to:
1 Perform an abbreviated physical examination of a dog.

Case Scenario and Candidate Tasks

Scene:
"Jack" is a 1-year-old male terrier presented for an exam prior to castration this afternoon. The owners report that Jack has no concerning issues.

Student Task:
You are to:
1 Perform a thorough, general physical exam.
2 Verbally report the TPR to your examiner (Please note: T has already been reported as normal by your technician).

Have your "technician" place "Jack" on the exam table and restrain "Jack" for you. Your "technician" (examiner) can only do exactly what you tell them to do.

Observe all standard safety procedures and protocols.

Jack's temperature has already been taken by your technician and is reported as normal.

It is important that you deliberately **perform each component of the examination, and also** verbally describe **what you are doing to the Examiner.**

If you are asked to "**PLEASE STOP the procedure**" you should immediately stop the activity and move away from the examining area.

Examiner's Information

Examiner's Information:

1 Prior to beginning the task, the student should be dressed in clean scrubs (lab coat over top is ideal) with professional closed toe shoes, and long hair tied back. If the student fails to be appropriately turned out for the station, they should be asked to change into appropriate attire and then return to perform the task. The clock will continue running until they are appropriately prepared and they will only have the time remaining when they return.

2 Examiner uses a double binaural stethoscope to confirm auscultation findings. Some leniency should be provided in determining heart rate and respiratory rate – the numbers the student provides should be close to what the examiner determined but may not be exact.

3 If the student fails to start the appropriate task or gets off task, then the examiner should state, "**Would you like to please re-read the scenario?**"

4 If the student endangers themselves, the animal, or the assistant at any time during the scenario, then tell them to, "**Please STOP what you are doing and move away from the exam procedure. Please remain at this station until you are asked to leave.**" (e.g. leaving a dog unattended on the table)

5 **The Examiner should examine the animal prior to the OSCE to know roughly what the dog's values for HR and RR are.**

At the end of the task, the examiner needs to:

1 The dog patient should be on the floor and waiting with the "technician" for the student to enter the room.

2 If a critical error occurs, please ask the student to remain in the station and ask the technician nearby to contact the course coordinator or clinical skills program director for assistance.

Station Checklist/Grading

The student should do the following:	Yes	No	Points
1 Make a visible effort to perform a distant examination before asking for the dog to be lifted onto the examination table.			1
2 Evaluates oral mucous membranes for color (pink) (lift lip, look at color).			1

The student should do the following:	**Yes**	**No**	**Points**
3 Evaluates oral mucous membranes for capillary refill time (lift lip, press finger into gingiva, release, time for color to return).			1
4 Examines both eyes.			1
5 Examines and looks into both ears.			1
6 Auscultates the <u>left</u> side of the chest – listening for at least 1–2 beats in more than one location (approximately over P – A – M valves).			1
7 Auscultates the heart on the <u>right</u> side of the chest at approximately the 3rd to 5th intercostal space mid thorax.			1
8 Assesses the heart rate <u>and</u> tells the examiner what the correct heart is *(must count and have accurate count)*.			1
9 Auscultate the lung fields by waiting and listening for at least one breath in each of 4 sites (cranioventral/caudodorsal; left and right) *(must listen to all 4 for points)*.			2
10 Assesses the respiratory rate <u>and</u> indicates the correct respiratory rate verbally to the examiner.			1
11 Palpates the abdomen: Use 2 hands for mid-size to large dog (1 hand acceptable in small dog or cat).			1
12 Adjusts hand position at least once during abdominal palpation – *not just going through the motions*.			1
13 Palpates <u>at least 2</u> sites for peripheral lymph nodes: • submandibular • pre-scapular • axillary • inguinal • popliteal			2
14 Performs the physical exam in a succinct manner, moving in a clear organized flow.			1
15 Does not startle dog by stopping/starting and/or jumping from head-to-tail-to-head, etc.			1
Total Points:			**17**
<u>Fatal Flaws:</u>		
If the student gravely endangers the animal, the assistant or themselves at any time during the scenario (e.g. puts dog on table and leaves unattended, mishandles animal and creates dangerous situation). If the student commits a critical error, tell the student to "Please <u>STOP</u> what you are doing and move away from the exam procedure. Please remain at this station until you are asked to leave." <u>A critical error MUST be called while the student is still in the station – This cannot be called after the student has already rotated</u>		

Global rating scale performance (*this will be used to calculate the passing/failing grades*):

Unable to Perform	Borderline	Satisfactory	Very Good	Excellent

Open comments

Station Equipment and Materials			
State the required equipment for this station:			
<u>Item</u>	<u>Amount</u>	<u>Brand</u>	<u>Specific Comments</u>
Binaural stethoscope	1/station		
Alcohol swabs (to clean stethoscope)	15/station		
Garbage can	1/station		
Calculator	1/station		
Hand sanitizer	1/station		
Dog treats – small container	1/station		
Exam table	1/station		
Clock	Visible to all stations		
Mats (for nonslip on table)	1/station		e.g. bath mat, rubber
State the required animals for this station:			
<u>Animal Required</u>	**<u>Amount</u>**	**<u>Specific Comments</u>**	
1 dog per exam station		Friendly and easy to handle	

Feedback from examiner:

Please share your opinion and experience, so we can improve this station for next year:

1. What worked well for this station?

   _____
   _____
   _____
   _____

2. Opportunities for improvement of this station:

   _____
   _____
   _____
   _____

3. Any additional information regarding pros and cons of each:

   a. Simulator_____
   b. Checklist/packet _____
   c. Supplies _____
   d. Time _____

Info to be shared with the students during the debriefing session after the end of the exams:

1. Top 3 most proficient steps observed:

   _____

   _____

   _____

   _____

2. Top 3 most deficient steps observed:

   _____

   _____

   _____

   _____

THANKS for helping us today!!

Surgical Towel Placement Rubric

Abi Taylor

NC State SimLab - Surgical Towel Placement Rubric

Demonstrate <u>4-corner surgical towel and towel clamp placement</u> **for an OVH procedure on a two-year-old female canine while remaining sterile (pretend that you are fully gowned and gloved).**

Dr. Abi Taylor

	Critical error (Requires deliberate practice)	Needs further practice (Requires deliberate practice)	Basic competence (Standards for performance)	Advanced (Evidence of exceeding standard)
Description	❑ Breaks sterility by: _____ _____ _____ ❑ Surgical field obscured ❑ Places towels incorrectly in a manner that would compromise surgical sterility ❑ Clamps would not adequately hold towels in place for procedure (multi-clamp error)	❑ Manipulates towels below level of surgical table ❑ Moves towel toward incision site after placement ❑ Surgical field partially obscured ❑ Places cranial drape at umbilicus instead of midway between umbilicus and xiphoid without correcting ❑ Places caudal drape too cranial to pubis without correcting ❑ Rolls hands outward when lifting from towels (vs. "lifting") ❑ Towel clamp misses skin ❑ Towel clamp skin "bite" too large ❑ Awkward hand and/or body movements ❑ Towels placed in incorrect order (far to near)	Completes toweling of the incision site and places towel clamps, within the time limit, using economy of motion and maintaining sterility.	Meets standards for performance, demonstrates exceptional efficiency and fluidity of movement; no awkwardness
Points	0	1	2	3

Veterinary Clinical Skills, First Edition. Edited by Emma K. Read, Matt R. Read, and Sarah Baillie.
© 2022 John Wiley & Sons, Inc. Published 2022 by John Wiley & Sons, Inc.
Companion website: www.wiley.com/go/read/veterinary

Pedicle Ligature (two-handed tie) Rubric

Abi Taylor

NC State SimLab - Pedicle Ligature (two-handed tie) Rubric

Demonstrate a <u>ligature tied using a two-handed technique</u> **on the vertical tubing immediately below the deepest clamp exactly as you would do for a dog with a fat ovarian pedicle. This is the first of the two ligatures you would place during a live spay.**

Dr. Abi Taylor

	Critical error (requires deliberate practice)	**Needs further practice** (requires deliberate practice)	**Basic competence** (standards for performance)	**Advanced** (evidence of exceeding standard)
Description	❑ Fails to place ligature on the correct side of the clamp ❑ Places 3 or fewer throws ❑ The ligature is loose	❑ No surgeon's throw ❑ Granny knot ❑ Fails to pull subsequent knots tight ❑ Significant hesitation/ awkwardness ❑ Fails to use "finger & thumb" technique ❑ Switching suture end hands between throws ❑ Reversed thumb and finger (crossed suture) ❑ Pulls up when tying ❑ Re-tries more than once	Completes the task of placing and tying hand-tie with good economy of motion Placement of knots is appropriate (4 throws on top of surgeon's throw/ friction knot) with minimal chance of failure The ligature is tight	Meets standards, demonstrates exceptional efficiency & fluidity of movement; no awkwardness
Points	**0**	**1**	**2**	**3**

Veterinary Clinical Skills, First Edition. Edited by Emma K. Read, Matt R. Read, and Sarah Baillie.
© 2022 John Wiley & Sons, Inc. Published 2022 by John Wiley & Sons, Inc.
Companion website: www.wiley.com/go/read/veterinary

Equine Handling & Restraint

Teresa Burns and Emma K. Read

College of Veterinary Medicine, The Ohio State University, Columbus, OH, USA

Learning Outcomes - This station will test the student's ability to:
1 Safely approach a horse in a stall
2 Apply a leather or nylon halter and lead rope
3 Lead the horse out of the stall
4 Make it go where the student wants to go (lead from the stall they are in and into/back out of the stall across.)

Case Scenario and Candidate Tasks

Scene:
You are handling a horse for a veterinarian at a clinic.

Student Task:
You are to:
1 **Approach** the horse in the stall.
2 Apply a leather or nylon **halter** and **lead rope.**
3 **Lead** the horse out of the stall.
4 Make it go where you want to go.

Student Information:
The examiner will ask you to lead the horse out of the stall, into the open stall across the alley, turn around, and then return into the original stall.
Use all of the handling and safety skills taught in your Clinical Skills sessions.
If you fail to start the appropriate task, then the examiner will state, **"Would you like to re-read the scenario?"**
If you are asked to **"PLEASE STOP the procedure,"** you should immediately stop the activity and move away from the examining area.

Veterinary Clinical Skills, First Edition. Edited by Emma K. Read, Matt R. Read, and Sarah Baillie.
© 2022 John Wiley & Sons, Inc. Published 2022 by John Wiley & Sons, Inc.
Companion website: www.wiley.com/go/read/veterinary

Examiner's Information:

1 The student should be dressed in clean coveralls and boots (or closed toed shoes). They should have long hair tied back. They should have no dangling jewelry. If the student fails to be appropriately turned out for the station, they should be asked to change appropriately and then do the task. The clock will continue until they are appropriately prepared and return.

2 The student is being asked to approach and halter the horse using a leather or nylon halter (one will accompany the horse). The student should organize the halter and lead rope such that the lead rope is safely collected in-hand and the halter is fully prepared prior to working with the horse. The student should greet the horse verbally and approach its left shoulder quietly (as indicated in the checklist) and allow the horse to sniff their hand or scratch the horse on the shoulder or neck. They should <u>offer</u> the nose part of the halter to the horse <u>before</u> placing it on the horse's nose. They should correctly hold the halter near the base of the poll strap and throatlatch loop while placing the horse's nose in the halter, then pushing the poll strap up over the poll and ears. They must not NOT flip it over the horse's poll causing surprise to the animal. They should correctly affix the halter buckle, then snap the lead rope onto correct ring of the halter and place the right hand within 10–20 cm of the halter shank but NOT directly on the snap. The student should place the remainder of the lead rope in their left hand and gather up the excess without coiling the rope around their hand.

3 The student should lead the horse by remaining on the left side (at the shoulder) and walk forward without looking back at the horse. The student should have confident body language that encourages the horse to move out and follow them. When approaching the object in the alleyway or turning in the stall, the horse should be pushed away from the student by a gentle push on the neck area or due to the proximity of the handler to the horse's left shoulder. Bringing the horse toward the handler as they turnaround is less desirable and considered less safe because the horse may run out over them.

4 If the student fails to start the appropriate task, then the examiner will state, **"Would you like to please re-read the scenario?"**

5 Dropping the lead rope or a portion of it into an area where the horse might step on it will be considered a **Critical Error**, as is wrapping any portion of the lead rope around the hand or other body part (both of these situations can result in injury to the student or horse). Standing in an unsafe position while leading or handling will also be considered a **Critical Error**.

6 If the candidate commits a **Critical Error**, they must be alerted before they leave the station. In the event of a **Critical Error**, the Examiner should say, **"Please STOP what you are doing and move away from the stocks. Please remain at this station until you are asked to leave."**

At the end of the task, the examiner needs to:

Take the halter and lead apart, ensure that the throatlatch loop is undone and open.

Ensure that the horse is usable for the next student. Alert support staff if horse is intractable or needs sedation – the horse can be exchanged for another horse and they can be removed from the exam.

The student should do the following:	<u>Yes</u>	<u>No</u>	Points
1 Prepares the halter by organizing it, ensuring the poll strap is open and safely arranging the lead rope in-hand before approaching the horse.			2
2 Greets the horse verbally or gently in a physical manner on or near the shoulder area.			1
3 Approaches the horse quietly from the left shoulder or left thorax area. (Note: Occasionally the horse will be standing in such a way that the candidate is safer to approach initially from the right shoulder or right thorax, and move the horse or place a lead rope on the horse's neck to move it. This will also receive a "yes" check mark.)			2

The student should do the following:	Yes	No	Points
4 Moves gently and slowly (e.g. allows the horse to sniff their hand or scratches the horse on the left side (or right as in the note in 3 above) of the neck or shoulder before beginning task).			1
5 <u>Offers</u> the nose part of the halter to the horse <u>before</u> placing it onto the horse's nose.			2
6 Correctly holds the halter near the base of the poll strap (crownpiece) and throatlatch loop ring while placing the horse's nose in the halter.			1
7 Correctly pushes the poll strap (crownpiece) up over the poll without pulling the halter into the horse's eyes.			1
8 Checks for 3–4 finger fit of the halter under the throatlatch and adjusts if necessary.			2
9 Attaches lead rope to the proper ring of the halter (circle ring and not D rings).			1
10 Places the right hand within 10–20 cm of the halter, but NOT directly on the snap.			1
11 Places the remainder of the lead rope in their left hand and gathers excess at all times to avoid tripping on it.			1
12 Candidate does not loop the excess lead rope around their hand. The excess should be laid back and forth in the candidate's hand.			3
13 Correctly and decisively, leads the horse forward and out of the stall from the horse's left (near) side.			1
14 Encourages the horse to move out freely by using confident body language.			3
15 Candidate leads the horse to the stall across the alley and turns around by asking the horse to move away from the handler.			3
16 Horse moves where candidate wants to go.			2
17 Leads horse back into original stall.			1
Total Points:			28

<u>Critical Errors:</u>

The student should not place themselves, the examiner, or the horse in imminent danger of getting seriously injured. <u>Critical Errors</u> include but are not limited to the following:

- Wrapping the lead rope around a hand or other body part.
- Dropping the end of the lead rope where the horse can step on it.
- Placing one's body in a position where they may get hurt easily.

Examiner asks you to **"Please STOP what you are doing and move away from the exam procedure, please remain at this station until you are asked to leave."**

<u>**A Critical Error MUST be called while the student is still in the station – This cannot be called after the student has already rotated.**</u>

Global rating scale performance (*this will be used to calculate the passing/failing grades*):

Unable to perform	Borderline	Satisfactory	Very good	Excellent

Open comments:

State the required equipment for this station:

Item	Amount	Brand	Specific comments
Halters that fit the horses below	1 per station		Ensure that they fit properly
Lead rope	1 per station		Same length and same snap please

State the required animals for this station:

Animal required	Amount	Specific comments
Tractable horses	8	Must catch easily and lead and back up easily to shoulder and/or nose pressure

Feedback from examiner:

Please share your opinion and experience so we can improve this station for next year:

1. What worked well for this station?
   _____
   _____
   _____
   _____

2. Opportunities for improvement of this station:
   _____
   _____
   _____
   _____

3. Any additional information regarding pros and cons of each:
   a. Simulator_____
   b. Checklist/packet _____
   c. Supplies _____
   d. Time _____

Info to be shared with the students during the debriefing session after the end of the exams:

1. Top 3 most proficient steps observed:
   _____
   _____
   _____
   _____

2. Top 3 most deficient steps observed:

_____

_____

_____

_____

THANKS for helping us today!!

Intramuscular Injection in a Canine Model

Julie Williamson

College of Veterinary Medicine, Lincoln Memorial University, Harrogate, TN, USA

Student task card
1 Show or tell the examiner how you would like them to restrain the dog.
2 Draw up 1 ml of room air.
3 Administer an intramuscular injection in the epaxial musculature.
4 Maintain proper sharps management throughout.
You have four minutes to complete this station.

Examiner information
You will examine the student performing the task and fill in the check list, as well as provide a global score of his/her performance.
If the student runs over time, instruct him/her to stop and move to the next station.

Required equipment		
ITEM	Amount	Specific comments
Canine intramuscular injection dog (Ikea)	4	2/station
3 cc syringes with 22 g 1" needles attached	100	
Sharps containers	4	2/station

Guidelines for accepted technique
Restraint: Student should demonstrate or tell the examiner to restrain the dog in standing recumbency.
Intramuscular injection: Student should palpate the dog's spine in between the ribs (cranial) and the wing of the ilium (caudal). Student should inject just off midline and insert at least half of the needle in order to enter the epaxial musculature. Student should aspirate before then injecting the air.
Sharps safety: Student should uncap the needle using his/her hands and not his/her teeth. After performing the intramuscular injection, student should either drop syringe/uncapped needle combo directly into the sharps container or recap the needle using a tabletop scoop technique.

Veterinary Clinical Skills, First Edition. Edited by Emma K. Read, Matt R. Read, and Sarah Baillie.
© 2022 John Wiley & Sons, Inc. Published 2022 by John Wiley & Sons, Inc.
Companion website: www.wiley.com/go/read/veterinary

Acceptable variations
Student may vary in which fingers he/she uses to operate the syringe. Some students will use the thumb to draw back on and then inject the plunger, while others will use the middle or ring finger to draw back and then switch to the thumb to inject. Numerous methods are acceptable as long as needle motion in the patient and sharps risk is minimized.
The student may either drop the syringe and uncapped needle combo directly into the sharps container or recap using a tabletop scoop technique, and then drop the syringe and capped needle into the sharps container.

Checklist			
	Student performed the following	**Yes (1)**	**No (0)**
1	Shows or tells examiner to hold dog in standing position		
2	Uncaps needle safely with hands		
3	Draws up 1 ml of air into the syringe		
4	Introduces needle alongside spine between last rib (cranially) and wing of the ilium (caudally) into the "epaxial musculature"		
5	Inserts needle at least halfway up to the hub		
6	Aspirates before then injecting air		
7	Does not shift hand around significantly on the syringe during procedure		
8	Does not recap needle OR recaps needle using tabletop scoop technique		
9	Drops needle and syringe into sharps container		

10	Global score					
	6	5	4	3	2	1
	Excellent	Good	Borderline satisfactory	Borderline unsatisfactory	Poor	Very poor

Mandatory station failure
Student does not complete the task within time allowed
Student performs a very superficial injection (i.e. just below the skin, clearly SQ) or inserts less than half of the needle into the model
Student stabs the model multiple times before inserting the needle for the injection
Student displays one serious flaw in sharps management (e.g. uncaps needle with teeth, leaves uncapped needle on the table, disconnects uncapped needle from syringe)

Anesthetic Machine Set-Up and Leak Testing

Matt R. Read[1] and Carolina Ricco Pereira[2]

[1] MedVet, Worthington, OH, USA
[2] College of Veterinary Medicine, The Ohio State University, Columbus, OH, USA

Learning Outcomes – This station will test the student's ability to:
Safely assemble and test an anesthetic machine and circle system breathing circuit.

Case Scenario and Student Tasks

Scene:
It is 7 a.m. on Monday morning. You are excited to be at work already and decide to get ready for the first procedure of the day: a 25-kg dog you have scheduled for a complete dental cleaning. Since your technician has not yet arrived, you decide to be helpful and set up the anesthetic machine and breathing circuit.

Student Task:
1 Set up the anesthetic machine and appropriate breathing circuit for this patient.
2 Perform a leak-test on the circuit.
3 Prepare the equipment so that a patient can be immediately connected to it.

Student Information:
If you are asked to **"PLEASE STOP the procedure"** you should immediately stop the activity and move away from the examining area, but wait in the station to move on to the next one.

Examiner's Information:
1 The student should set up a circle breathing system and pressure test it.
2 If the student leaves the pop-off valve closed after testing the circuit or if the student takes their thumb off the end of the circuit THEN re-opens the pop-off valve after testing for leaks (i.e. they don't open valve to test its function before removing thumb), then a **Critical Error** must be called. You should say **"Please STOP what you are doing and move away from the exam procedure. Please remain in this station until you are asked to rotate onwards."**

Veterinary Clinical Skills, First Edition. Edited by Emma K. Read, Matt R. Read, and Sarah Baillie.
© 2022 John Wiley & Sons, Inc. Published 2022 by John Wiley & Sons, Inc.
Companion website: www.wiley.com/go/read/veterinary

At the end of the station, the examiner needs to:
1 Take the components of the anesthesia machine apart and return it to the state in which it was at the start of the station.
2 Make sure all of the components are displayed and available for the next student to pick from.

SA Anesthesia Station Checklist/Grading

The student should do the following:	Yes	No	Points:
1 Attach the oxygen supply hose (green) to the ceiling mount.			1
2 Attach scavenge hose (purple) to ceiling mount.			1
3 Check isoflurane level in vaporizer to make sure there is an adequate level for use.			1
4 Attach circle system breathing circuit to the machine.			1
5 Attach reservoir bag to machine.			1
6 Close pop-off valve. (Steps 6, 7, and 8 can be in any order)			2
7 Turn on oxygen flowmeter or activate the flush valve.			2
8 Occlude the end of the breathing circuit with their thumb/hand/etc.			2
9 Allow reservoir bag to fill with oxygen while watching circuit pressure gauge.			1
10 Turn off the oxygen flowmeter or stop using the flush when the pressure is between 30 and 40 cm H_2O.			2
11 Hold this pressure and wait 5–10 seconds to check for leaks in the system (the circuit pressure will drop if there is a leak).			1
12 After test, open pop-off valve completely so reservoir bag expels contents.			3
13 After pop-off valve opened, remove thumb from circuit (THIS CAN ONLY BE DONE AFTER THE POP-OFF VALVE HAS ALREADY BEEN OPENED IN STEP 12!!)			3
Total Points:			**21**
Critical Errors: **Leaves Pop-off valve closed after testing circuit.** **Takes thumb off the end of the circuit THEN re-opens the pop-off valve after testing for leaks (i.e. they don't open valve to test its function before removing thumb).**	Yes	No	

Global rating scale performance (*this will be used to calculate the passing/failing grades*):

Unable to perform	Borderline	Satisfactory	Very good	Excellent

Open comments:

Station equipment and materials

State the required equipment for this station (insert more lines if needed):			
Item	**Amount**	**Brand**	**Specific comments**
Small animal anesthetic machine	1 per station		
Circle system circuit	1 per station		
2L reservoir bag	1 per station		

Feedback from examiner:

Please share your opinion and experience so we can improve this station for next year:

1. What worked well for this station?

2. Opportunities for improvement of this station:

3. Any additional information regarding pros and cons of each:
   a. Simulator_____
   b. Checklist/packet _____
   c. Supplies _____
   d. Time _____

Info to be shared with the students during the debriefing session after the end of the exams:

1. Top 3 most proficient steps observed:

2. Top 3 most deficient steps observed:

THANKS for helping us today!!

Appendix 2

Recipes for Making Clinical Skills Models

The following recipes have been provided by clinical skills teams to illustrate how to make a range of simple models for use in teaching. Each recipe follows a standardized template:

- Model name
- Ingredients for making the model and where to source the materials
- Steps for making the model
- Tips for making and using the model
- Supporting learning resources for use when teaching/learning with the model
- References

All the model recipes are available with the images in color on the companion website (www.wiley.com/go/read/veterinary).

The models in this appendix are:

Canine castration model
Lindsey Ramirez, Megan Preston, Julie Hunt

Dental scaling model
Rachel Harris, Andrew Gardiner, Rachel Lumbis

Endotracheal intubation model
Maire O'Reilly

Equine abdominocentesis model
Catherine May, Catherine Werners, Keshia John, Sarah Baillie, Emma Read

Canine leg with cephalic vein model
Lissann Wolfe

Silicone skin suturing model
Marc Dilly

SimSpay model
Rikke Langebæk

Surgical prep model
Jean-Yin Tan and Alfredo Romero

Tea towel suturing model
Alison Catterall

Veterinary Clinical Skills, First Edition. Edited by Emma K. Read, Matt R. Read, and Sarah Baillie.
© 2022 John Wiley & Sons, Inc. Published 2022 by John Wiley & Sons, Inc.
Companion website: www.wiley.com/go/read/veterinary

Canine Castration Model

Lindsey Ramirez, Megan Preston, and Julie Hunt

College of Veterinary Medicine, Lincoln Memorial University, Harrogate, TN, USA

Ingredients for making the model	Where to source the materials & notes
Canine testicle mold box (76.2 cm × 31.1 cm × 9.8 cm) Constructed of 19-mm thick vinyl-laminated plywood and wood screws	This size mold box will create 10 testicles
Zinc-free modeling clay	
Plastic drinking straws	
Drill & drill bits (9.5, 3.2, 6.4 mm hole punch)	
Wire	Gauge of wire should fit through the plastic drinking straws
Hot glue gun & glue sticks	
Wooden paint sticks (24.5 cm long) × 10	Use 9.5 mm drill bit to pre-drill holes 7.6 cm & 20.3.2 mm from the top
Wooden dowel rods (9.5 mm × 5.1 cm long) × 20	
Brass nuts × 6	
Mold Star 15 Silicone Mold Rubber	Source: Smooth-On, Inc. (Macungie, PA)
Ecoflex 00–30 Platinum Cure Silicone Rubber	Source: Smooth-On, Inc. (Macungie, PA)
Silc Pig Red Silicone Pigment 59 ml	Source: Smooth-On, Inc. (Macungie, PA)
Silc Pig Flesh Silicone Pigment 59 ml	Source: Smooth-On, Inc. (Macungie, PA)
Clear square plastic box with lid (15.24 cm × 15.24 cm × 2.54 cm)	Esslinger.com
12.7 mm unslotted white rapid assembly post & screw	Product Components Corporation (Martinez, CA)

Veterinary Clinical Skills, First Edition. Edited by Emma K. Read, Matt R. Read, and Sarah Baillie.
© 2022 John Wiley & Sons, Inc. Published 2022 by John Wiley & Sons, Inc.
Companion website: www.wiley.com/go/read/veterinary

Ingredients for making the model	Where to source the materials & notes
Ease Release 200	Source: Smooth-On, Inc. (Macungie, PA)
Parafilm "M" laboratory film	
Household iron (laundry)	
Vacuum pump with tubing hose	
60 ml syringe	
Condoms (black or dark in color) × 2	
Apricot power mesh (15.24 cm × 15.24 cm) 80% nylon/20% spandex	Theengineerguy.com
Small rubber bands × 2	
#10 scalpel & blade	
Lubricating jelly	

Steps for Making the Model

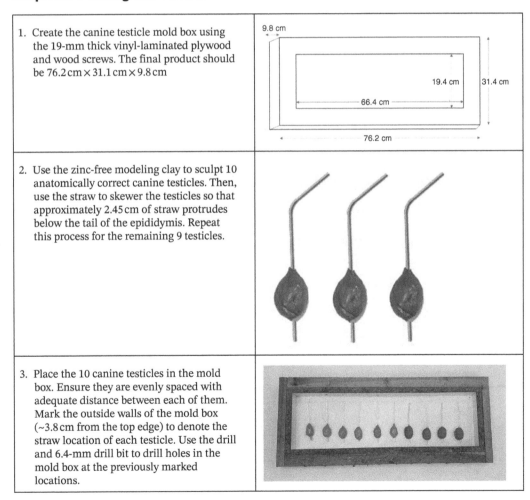

1. Create the canine testicle mold box using the 19-mm thick vinyl-laminated plywood and wood screws. The final product should be 76.2 cm × 31.1 cm × 9.8 cm

2. Use the zinc-free modeling clay to sculpt 10 anatomically correct canine testicles. Then, use the straw to skewer the testicles so that approximately 2.45 cm of straw protrudes below the tail of the epididymis. Repeat this process for the remaining 9 testicles.

3. Place the 10 canine testicles in the mold box. Ensure they are evenly spaced with adequate distance between each of them. Mark the outside walls of the mold box (~3.8 cm from the top edge) to denote the straw location of each testicle. Use the drill and 6.4-mm drill bit to drill holes in the mold box at the previously marked locations.

4. Feed the wire through the drilled hole on the mold box and the straw of the testicle. The wire will exit through the mold box at the short end of the straw. Secure each end of wire to the mold box to suspend the testicles in the box. Repeat this step for the remaining 9 testicles. Then, use the hot glue gun to fill in each hole around the wire (this ensures Mold Star will not leak out).

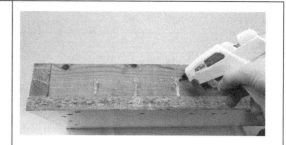

5. Spray the canine testicles and mold box with Ease Release 200. Mix enough Mold Star 15 to fill the mold box halfway up the side of the canine testicle. Slowly pour the Mold Star 15 into one corner of the box and allow it to self-level. When the Mold Star 15 becomes tacky, drop a pair of brass nuts into the space between the testicles, ensuring there is a pair on the left, right, and middle of the mold box. Allow the mold to cure overnight.

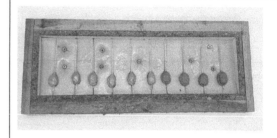

6. Insert the dowel rods into the predrilled holes of the paint sticks. Remove the brass nuts from the mold. Spray the testicles, cured mold, paint sticks, and dowel rods with Ease Release 200. Center the paint sticks and dowel rods over the top of each testicle and use weight to secure them down. Use Mold Star 15 to fill the rest of the mold box by slowly pouring into one corner of the box and allow it to self-level. Allow the mold to cure overnight.

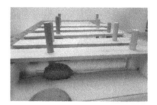

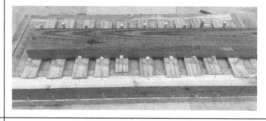

7. Locate seam of mold and carefully separate the top from the bottom. Remove clay testicles by cutting the suspension wire close to the inside of the mold frame to reveal a negative impression of 10 canine testicles with spermatic cords.

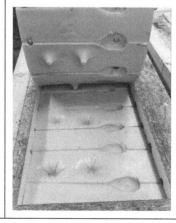

8. Spray inside of mold generously with Ease Release 200 and replace the top by aligning the indentations made by the weight of the brass nuts. Using a 60-ml syringe, apply red tinted silicone into one opening while using a pump to suck air out of its adjacent opening. This ensures silicone fills the mold entirely and aids in avoiding air bubbles. Repeat for all 10 testicles. Allow four hours for silicone to cure.

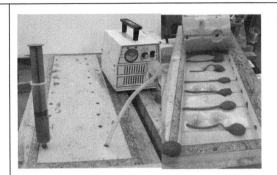

9. The base of the model is created in a similar fashion as the testicles using the 15.24 cm × 15.24 cm clear plastic box. Use a straw to create a hole in the clay on each side of the preputial area equal distance apart.

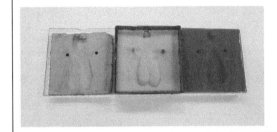

10. The skin is created by pouring 60 ml of flesh tinted silicone into the 15.24 cm × 15.24 cm clear plastic box. Power Mesh (15.24 cm × 15.24 cm) is placed on top and allowed to sink into the wet silicone. Allow four hours for silicone to cure.

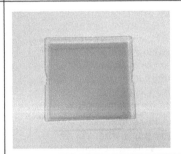

11. Cut parafilm into 33 cm × 10.2 cm strips. Lay 2 pieces on top of each other (parafilm side touching) and use the side of an iron to melt a thin line in the center to bond the pieces together, creating the median raphe.

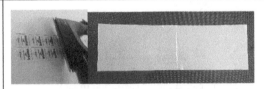

12. Using the 6.4-mm hole punch drill bit, create evenly spaced openings in the model base to allow insertion of white rapid assembly posts that will secure skin to base.

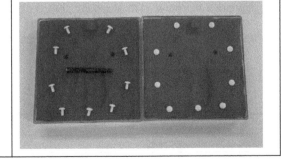

13. Open a condom, insert testicle, and place a rubber band at the base of the testicle. Place the parafilm on the model base and align the seam with the prepuce. Open the top flap of parafilm and make a small cut over the hole in the base. Thread the top of the condom through the hole and tuck it under the base. Lay the testicle in the impression in the mold. Repeat for the other side.

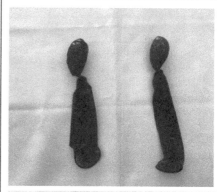

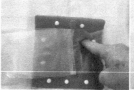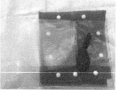

14. Apply a thin layer of lubricating jelly to the top of both testicles. Cover both testicles with the top layer of parafilm. Tuck excess parafilm under the base and place inside the 15.24 cm × 15.24 cm clear plastic box. Using the scalpel blade, make small incisions in the parafilm over the white rapid assembly posts and secure it under the posts.

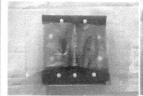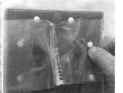

15. Lay the 15.24 cm × 15.24 cm silicone skin on the model. Make tiny incisions in the skin to secure it over the white rapid assembly posts.

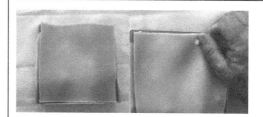

16. The completed canine castration model can be used to simulate a scrotal castration, or a pre-scrotal castration if the testicles are pushed forward into the pre-scrotal space.

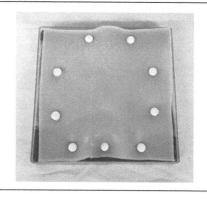

Reference

Hunt, J. A., Heydenburg, M., Kelly, C. K., et al. 2020. Development and validation of a canine castration model and rubric. *J Vet Med Educ*, 47, 1, 78–90.doi: https://doi.org/10.3138/ jvme.1117-158r1.

Dental Scaling Model

Rachel Harris[1], Andrew Gardiner[2], and Rachel Lumbis[3]

[1] Bristol Veterinary School, University of Bristol, Bristol, United Kingdom
[2] Royal (Dick) School of Veterinary Studies, University of Edinburgh, Scotland, United Kingdom
[3] Royal Veterinary College, Hatfield, United Kingdom

Ingredients for making the model	Where to source the materials
A white ceramic tile (150×150 mm)	Home improvements store
Dentition stencil	From Stencil Studio at: info@thestencilstudio.com Quote Ref: S – Teeth
Fine-tipped permanent marker pen	
Dental chart (laminated sheet)	Print a canine dental chart used in the clinic
Red insulation/electrical tape (19 mm)	Hardware store or online
Polyfilla	Preferably use a quick drying Polyfilla
Spreader (wooden stirrer)	
Red nail polish	N.B. Instead of standard nail varnish use a gel nail varnish (e.g. Maybelline Forever Strong Gel 06 Deep Red Nail Polish) as this does not wash off.
Scissors	
Incontinence sheet (to work on)	

Veterinary Clinical Skills, First Edition. Edited by Emma K. Read, Matt R. Read, and Sarah Baillie.
© 2022 John Wiley & Sons, Inc. Published 2022 by John Wiley & Sons, Inc.
Companion website: www.wiley.com/go/read/veterinary

Steps for Making the Model

Steps	
1. The model represents two quadrants of a dog's mouth. Turn the ceramic tile so it makes a diamond shape on the sheet (pad) on the table and place the stencil over it. Use a small piece of insulating tape to secure the stencil in place.	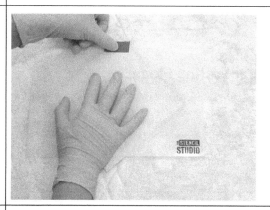
2. Using the black fine-tipped permanent marker pen, draw the outline of the teeth on the tile using the stencil to produce a lateral (buccal) view. N.B. There is a line connecting the teeth, which represents the root/crown junction. This normally lies below the gum line.	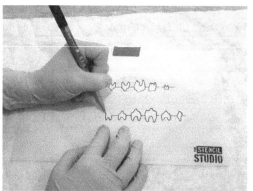
3. Once the marker has dried (approximately one to two minutes), remove the tape and the stencil. At this point, students making the model can be asked to identify which quadrants of a dog's mouth the stencil represents? If unsure, the student should check the canine dental chart (laminated sheet) provided.	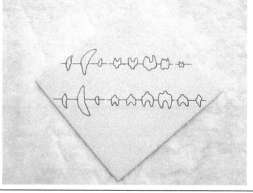
4. N.B. When extracting teeth, it is important to know the number of roots for each tooth. However, some of the roots are not clearly outlined on the stencil. Therefore, refer to the dental chart to check the number of roots for each individual tooth and then, for the relevant teeth, draw these roots on the tile using the fine-tipped marker pen.	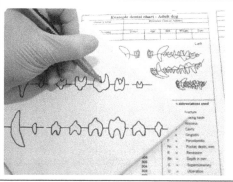

Steps	
5. Number the teeth according to the modified Triadan system (which is used across species, not just for dogs). If necessary, use the dental chart as a reference.	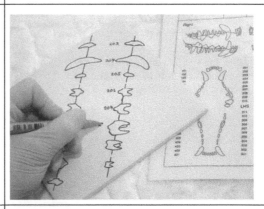
6. Next, create a pressure test square using the fine-tipped marker pen to draw a square (approximately $2\,cm^2$) in a free corner of the tile. This square is used for students to practice initially to hold the dental scaling handpiece correctly and to learn how to apply an appropriate amount of pressure.	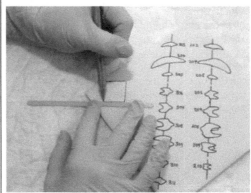
7. Fill in the square with a thin layer of nail varnish.	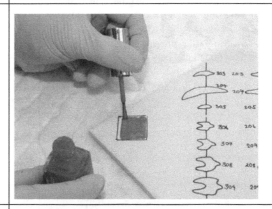
8. While waiting for the nail varnish to dry, apply a small amount of Polyfilla to the wooden spreader. The Polyfilla represents the calculus. Apply a layer over the surface of each tooth, trying to stay within the tooth outline. Apply the Polyfilla near the root/crown junction as this will mimic subgingival calculus once the gum line is in place.	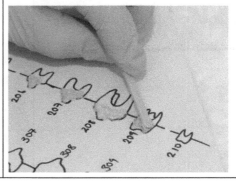

Steps	
9. Once the nail varnish is dry, apply a thin layer of Polyfilla over the pressure test square. Allow the Polyfilla on the teeth to dry (approximately 5–10 minutes) and then move on to the next step.	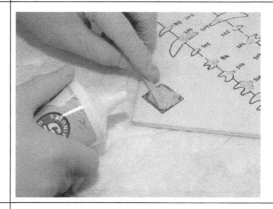
10. When performing a dental scale, quite often calculus is found in the gingival sulcus (below the gum line). Measure and cut a length of the red tape for the gum (it needs to be long enough to run diagonally from one edge of the tile to the other along the line of the root-crown junction).	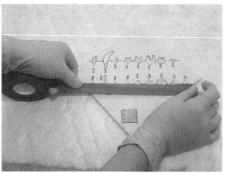
11. Create a small fold in the tape. This will form a "lip" when the tape is placed on the tile against the line of the teeth. This "lip" will represent the gingival sulcus (small gap between the tooth and the gingival tissue).	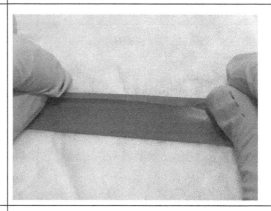
12. The tape should be placed such that it covers the roots of the teeth and some of the calculus near the root-crown junction, i.e. at a level that ensures some calculus (Polyfilla) is in the gingival sulcus.	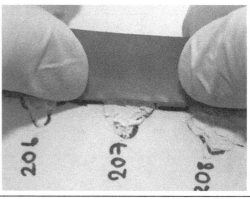

Steps	
13. Lay a piece of tape along the line of the teeth for the maxilla and another piece for the mandible. The model should now be placed to one side to allow the Polyfilla to completely dry.	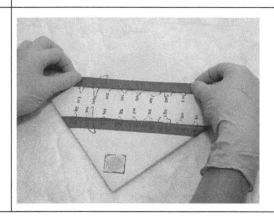

Supporting learning resources for use when teaching/learning with the model

Instruction booklet for students, including showing how to make the model: www.bristol.ac.uk/media-library/sites/vetscience/documents/clinical-skills/Dental%20Scaling.pdf

Acknowledgments

The original version of the model was created by Rachel Lumbis as part of her MSc project, it was modified by Andrew Gardiner and the current version was adapted by Rachel Harris.

Reference

Lumbis, R., Gregory, S., Baillie, S. 2012. Evaluation of a dental model for training veterinary students. *J Vet Med Educ*, 39, 2, 128–135. https://doi.org/10.3138/jvme.1011.108R

Endotracheal Intubation Model

Maire O'Reilly

University College Dublin, Dublin, Ireland

Ingredients for making the model	Where to source the materials & notes
• **Mouth, tongue, pharynx, larynx**: Foam dressing 12 cm × 12 cm	Wound dressing suppliers, e.g. Renofoam FOI4 20 cm × 20 cm, out of date hospital stock
• **Trachea:** Corrugated tubing 20 cm long 2.5 cm diameter	Standard anesthetic scavenging tubing
• **Lung:** Anesthetic rebreathing bag 2l or less	Balloon as an alternative choice
• **Esophagus** – Bicycle inner tube 20 cm long 3–4 cm diameter	Bicycle shop
• Marker pen	
• Zinc oxide tape 2.5 cm wide	Secures "trachea" to larynx
• Superglue	Reinforcement
• Cohesive bandage	Vetwrap
• Needle/thread	Suture on noncutting needle to over sew the attached pieces and the tongue
• Wide pen/pencil	
• Scissors and scalpel blade	Size 15 scalpel blade
• Soft toy dog	IKEA

Veterinary Clinical Skills, First Edition. Edited by Emma K. Read, Matt R. Read, and Sarah Baillie.
© 2022 John Wiley & Sons, Inc. Published 2022 by John Wiley & Sons, Inc.
Companion website: www.wiley.com/go/read/veterinary

Steps for Making the Model

1 Cut out a 12 cm × 12 cm piece of foam dressing.

2 On the inside of this piece:
- Mark with pen as illustrated
- Mark the larynx in the center as a 2.5-cm diameter circle or mark the outline against the actual corrugated tubing (the trachea)

3 Cut along the dark-gray dashed lines

Leave the larynx opening <u>uncut,</u> until the whole model is assembled – see step 16

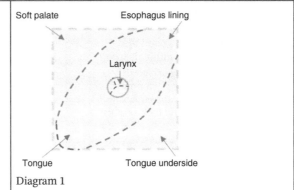

Diagram 1

Assemble model

4 Sew the tubing to the tongue

5 Place strips of zinc oxide tape between the tongue and trachea – continue around the full circle

6 While placing the zinc oxide tape, put a dab of glue on each sticky surface

7 Allow this assembly to dry

Diagram 2

8 Align the esophagus tubing (bicycle inner tube) against the trachea tubing

9 Push the esophagus lining (see Diagram 1) by "coning" the material and pushing it down the inside surface of the esophagus

10 Roll back the lining and hold securely at the top while dabbing glue on the esophagus tubing – push esophagus lining back in place

11 Glue the soft palate (Diagram 1) piece in the same way, down into the esophagus tubing, directly opposite to the esophagus lining piece – overlap to form esophagus lining

12 Place a suitably wide pen into the esophagus

13 Wrap with Vetwrap, as illustrated and allow the glue to dry – this keeps the assembly from loosening

Remove the pen when dry

14 Over sew the side of the tongue and soft palate pieces together – as the illustration – how much to sew depends on the size of your model. Cut the larynx anatomy carefully – dotted lines – with the size 15 blade (Diagram 1)

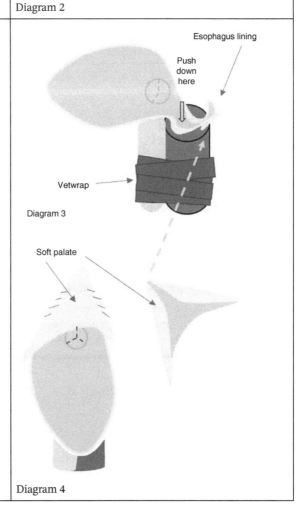

Diagram 3

Diagram 4

Assemble the model within the dog

15 Tape the rebreathing bag to the scavenging tubing at a point that positions it correctly within the chest

- The underside tongue piece (Diagram 1) can be sewn now if required. Sew with the pink sides together, reverse and tuck surplus under the dog mouth material (not essential but does reinforce the tongue)

16 Insert the finished assembly into the IKEA dog by unpicking the tongue and pushing the whole into the dog. Maneuver it in place from the outside or unpick part of the midline chest sewing and sew on Velcro fastening for access – recommended

17 Sew the soft palate piece (see Diagram 1) to the dog mouth roof material – judge the position of the larynx before sewing

18 Further sewing at the mouth opening depends on the dog you have used. The assembly can be left loose or anchor the model by sewing at the sides – allow for desired movement

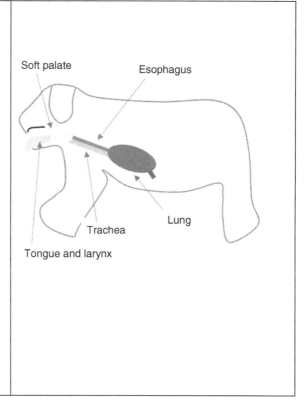

Top Tips for Making and Using the Model

- The IKEA Golden Gossig model has been used for this pattern. Other similar toy dogs with a mouth and tongue configuration are equally suitable.
- It is possible to make the model using out of date and used materials from left over hospital stock.
- Used bicycle inner tube can be obtained free from a bicycle repair shop (recycle!).
- When intubated, an Ambu bag facilitates the simulation during teaching and can be used to demonstrate that the tube is in the correct place as the lungs and chest expand
- When intubated his model can attach to an anesthetic machine.

Suggested additions to the model:

- Mold a maxilla using malleable material – like casting bandage – and fit into the head.
- A nasogastric tube can be added to the finished model – open the nares and track down to the pharynx – sew/glue a soft tubing (e.g. suction unit tubing) of suitable diameter from one nostril to a point on the soft palate piece leading into the esophagus.
- A nasal oxygen line can be added from the second nostril, sew/glue tubing (e.g. old ET tube) of suitable diameter from the nostril further to the medial canthus of that eye.

Supporting learning resources for use when teaching/ learning with the model

Endotracheal intubation instruction booklet: http://www.bristol.ac.uk/vet-school/research/comparative-clinical/veterinary-education/clinical-skills-booklets/anaesthesia-fluid-therapy/

Reference

Harris, R., O'Reilly, M., Baillie, S. 2020. Evaluation of an endotracheal intubation model and practical for training veterinary nursing students. *Vet Nurs J*, 35, 2, 42–45. DOI: https://doi.org/10.1080/17415349.2019.1697631.

Equine Abdominocentesis Model

Catherine May[1], Catherine Werners[2], Keshia John[2], Sarah Baillie[3], and Emma K. Read[4]

[1] Faculty of Veterinary Science, University of Pretoria, Pretoria, South Africa
[2] School of Veterinary Medicine, St. George's University, Grenada, West Indies
[3] Bristol Veterinary School, Bristol, United Kingdom
[4] College of Veterinary Medicine, The Ohio State University, Columbus, OH, USA

Ingredients for making the model	Where to source the materials
• Plastic barrel 48 gallon (220 liters) with lid	Can be ordered online, e.g. from Amazon
• Wooden "legs" × 4; crossbeams × 4 (wooden boards approx. 4" × 1.75" or 10 cm × 3 cm)	Hardware store
• Screws to attach crossbeams to legs	Hardware store
• Bolts × 8 (½" × 2¼" long or 1.2 cm × 6 cm) to attach legs to barrel	Hardware store
• Circular cutter or jigsaw	
• Brown paint (or whatever color you want your horse to be!)	Hardware store
• Sturdy plastic tub or plastic drainage piping approx. 4.5" (11 cm) diameter and cut to 5–6" (13–15 cm) tall	Food container or kitchen storage tub Plastic drainage pipe from hardware store
• Ecoflex 00–20 silicon (A & B)	https://www.smooth-on.com/
• Pigment (pink)	https://www.smooth-on.com/
• Wooden stick/stirrer	E.g. a coffee stirrer or tongue depressor
• Large (old) dinner plate	
• Baby powder	Pharmacy
• Cable tie (approx. 18" or 45 cm long)	Hardware store
• Red food coloring	Supermarket
• Vinyl glove	Supermarket

N.B. Sizes and measurement conversions from imperial to metric are approximate.

Steps for Making the Model

1. Remove the lid from the barrel. Use a jigsaw or circular cutter to cut an approximately 5–5.5″ (13–14 cm) diameter hole in the center of one side of the barrel. This is where the insert (see Step 3) is placed for the abdominocentesis.	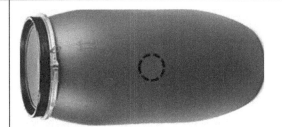
2. Make the wooden frame. Attach the four crossbeams between the legs for extra sturdiness. Bolt the legs to the barrel ensuring that the abdominocentesis hole is at the lowest point and the "belly" is at a suitable height, e.g. approximately 38″ (1 m) from the ground Paint the model.	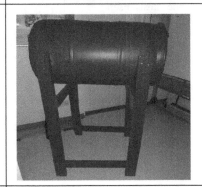
3. Make the abdominocentesis insert. Check the diameter of the tub or pipe is at least ½″ (1 cm) smaller than the hole in the barrel. Cut the plastic piping at 5–6″ (13–15 cm). Or cut the bottom off the sturdy plastic tub.	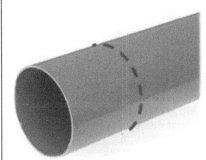
4. Make the abdominal wall for the abdominocentesis. Mix approximately 100 ml of Ecoflex silicon B with 10–15 drops of pink pigment. Stir with the wooden stick to make sure the color is evenly distributed. Add approximately 100 ml of Ecoflex silicon A to B and mix with the stirrer.	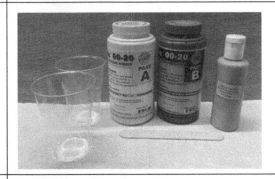
5. Pour silicon onto a large dinner plate. Remove (pop) any bubbles. Ensure the plate is level using a spirit level. Leave to set (several hours or overnight). Dust the surface of the dry silicon with baby powder (removes sticky feel).	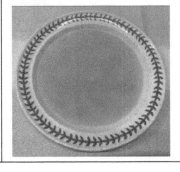

6. Place the silicon over the end of the tub (left photo) or pipe (right photo) and secure with a cable tie.	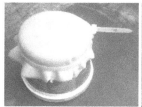 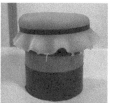
7. Secure the abdominocentesis insert into the circular hole in the barrel. Ensure it is firmly wedged and will not move using some padding, e.g. foam or wadding, between the barrel and the insert. If it is necessary to hold the insert more securely, screw 4 hooks into the inside of the plastic drum. Tie string to the hooks; pass the string over the insert to hold it in place.	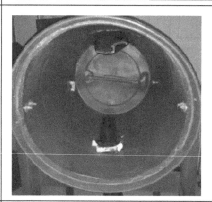

8. To make the abdominal fluid, add a few drops of red food coloring to approx. ½ pint or 200 ml of water.
  a. Pour into the tub insert. Or
  b. Pour into a vinyl glove and tie the glove with string or a cable tie.
Place the glove in the insert, push in firmly and weigh down with an object to make good contact with the silicon. After using the model, either a) remove the insert and pour out the liquid or b) remove the glove and dry the inside of the insert.
	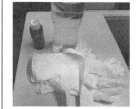 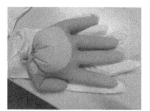

9. The finished model. An optional tail and head can be added.	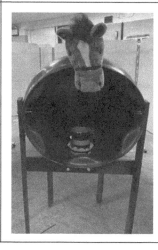

Top Tips for Making and Using the Model

- Ensure the wood used for the legs is sturdy enough and can carry the weight of the barrel. Always use the cross beams and ensure the bolts are secure to avoid the model rocking when in use. Use treated wood and paint model to avoid rot.
- To avoid leaks, remove the liquid and/or replace the glove with "blood" after each use.
- As an alternative to silicon, the abdominal wall can be made from neoprene.
- The barrel is used as a cheap alternative to buying a full size horse to make the model. A full size horse model could be adapted. However, access to the inside will need to be created, and this will require the use of cutting equipment that is suitable for the model material, e.g. fiberglass. Do not attempt without the correct equipment.

Acknowledgments

The carpentry team at SGU for making the model.

Dr. Emma Read developed the original idea with an insert in a full-size model horse. Dr. Sarah Baillie developed the version using the barrel.

Canine Leg with Cephalic Vein Model

Lissann Wolfe

School of Veterinary Medicine, College of Medical, Veterinary & Life Sciences, University of Glasgow, Glasgow, United Kingdom

Ingredients for making the model	Where to source the materials
• MDF (medium-density fiber) board 18 mm thick	Hardware store
• Rubber tubing 5 mm Versilon (24 m × 5 mm diameter; 1.5 mm wall thickness)	Lab supplies company (VWR) https://uk.vwr.com/store/product/577395/tubing-rubber-versilontm-gs
• Metal hook	Hardware store
• 500–1000 ml fluid bag	Veterinary wholesaler
• Food coloring red + blue	Supermarket
• Foam pipe approx. 4–5 cm diameter (used for insulation)	Hardware Store
• Cohesive bandage	Veterinary wholesaler
• Soffban 5 cm	Veterinary wholesaler
• 14 g × 1.5″ needle	Veterinary wholesaler
• Standard giving set	Veterinary wholesaler

Veterinary Clinical Skills, First Edition. Edited by Emma K. Read, Matt R. Read, and Sarah Baillie.
© 2022 John Wiley & Sons, Inc. Published 2022 by John Wiley & Sons, Inc.
Companion website: www.wiley.com/go/read/veterinary

Steps for Making the Model

Cut MDF sheets to size and assemble. • Vertical panel 76 cm × 15 cm • Horizontal panel 61 cm × 5 cm • Triangular block – 6 cm × 5 cm × 8 cm • Cut 5 cm hole in vertical panel approx. 24 cm from base • Screw the hook in near the top of the back of the vertical panel. They can be painted any color of choice before assembly.	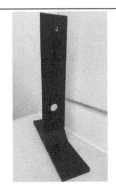
Inject fluid bag with sufficient food coloring to turn fluid a dark red. This will be the fake blood. You will require a standard giving set and 14 g × 1.5″ needle.	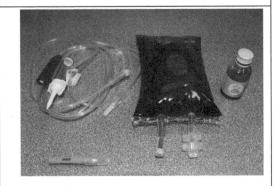
Cut foam piping to approx. 30 cm length. Cut rubber tubing to approx. 45 cm length.	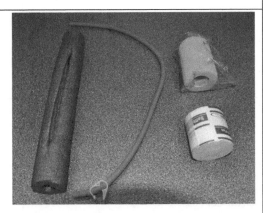
Attach the clamp from a used giving set to the end of the tubing opposite from the padded end.	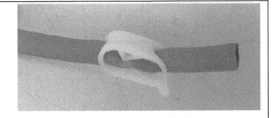

Pierce 2 holes at either end of the foam pipe and feed through red tubing so that a significant length sits along the outside of the foam pipe. This will be the cephalic vein.	
Wrap a small amount of 5 cm Soffban around one end of the foam piping.	
Cover entire length of foam piping with cohesive bandaging.	
Pass the covered foam pipe through the 5 cm hole in the vertical part of the stand. It should fit tightly with little movement. Additional padding can be added if too loose. Make sure the rubber tubing is palpable and in the center facing the user.	
Insert the spike on the fluid chamber into the opposite end of the rubber tubing to the one with the clamp.	
Attach the 14 g needle to the end of the giving set.	
Insert the 14 g needle into the injection port on the fluid bag.	

Hang the bag on the hook at the back of the model. Run the fluid through into a small bowl to fill the tubing with the fake blood. Once fully run through, close the clamp at the end of the rubber tubing. Ensure the regulator and clamp on giving set remain open.	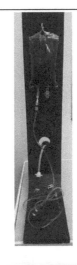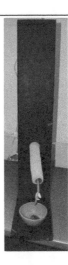
The finished model can be used for IV access and will give a satisfying flashback of "blood" when the needle or catheter is correctly placed in the vein.	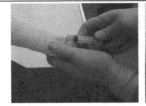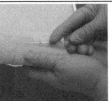

Tips for Making and Using the Model

- Adding a few drops of blue food dye helps make the fluid a darker red.
- When inserting the spike on the fluid chamber of the giving set into the tubing, lubricating the spike with water will allow for ease of insertion.
- If flashback is not achieved and the needle or catheter is definitely within the "vein," there may be a bubble within the tubing. To clear run fluid through into a bowl as before.

- Close the regulator and the clamp at the back of the model when not in use – this will prevent leakage from needle punctures.
- The rubber tubing is robust and will last quite a long time without significant leakage. When too damaged from repeated punctures replace with a new piece of rubber tubing.
- We use expired IV fluids for this model, which is typically glucose saline (although any IV fluid can be used). It is likely to grow fungus etc. within a couple of weeks and then needs to be replaced.
- The model can be stabilized by clamping it to a table or bench top, e.g. with a G clamp.

Silicone Skin Suturing Model

Marc Dilly

Faculty of Veterinary Medicine, Justus Liebig University Giessen, Giessen, Germany

Ingredients for making the model	Where to source the materials
• (Wooden) Mold	Do-it-yourself store
• Ecoflex 00-20 (silicone component A & B)	https://www.smooth-on.com/
• Pigments (fleshtone, red)	https://www.smooth-on.com/
• Powermesh, 135 × 120 mm	https://www.kaupo.de/shop/VAKUUMHAUBEN-SYSTEM/WHITE-POWER-MESH.html
• Foam material	Do-it-yourself store
• (Baby-)Powder	Drugstore

Steps for Making the Model

Steps	
1 Make the casting mold from wood (approximately 14.5 cm × 13 cm) with synthetic leather on the base (for an authentic look/texture of the skin) i.e. check its level using a spirit-level. 2 Mix approximately 25 ml of silicone component-B with a few drops of "skin" pink pigment. Stir with a wooden lollypop stick or coffee stirrer (picture A). 3 Add approximately 25 ml of silicone component-A to component-B and mix. 4 Fill the casting mold with the mixture of silicone and wait for approximately 60 minutes. 5 Once the first layer has set, repeat steps 2 and 3 for the second layer using red pigment. 6 Place the mesh on top of the first layer and use a paint-brush to spread a thin layer of the red silicone over the mesh (picture B shows the white mesh in place and the painting with red silicone in progress). 7 Eliminate any bubbles before filling the mold with the remaining red silicone (picture C). 8 The foam material (in the bottom right hand corner of photos B & C) is immediately placed on top of the second layer of silicone and held in place, e.g. with a wooden block. 9 Wait for approximately 180 minutes for the model to set. 10 Remove the suture pad from the casting mold and use a brush to lightly dust some powder on the skin surface to remove the slightly "sticky" feel.	(a) 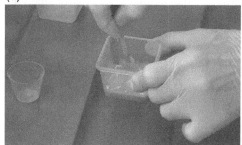 (b) 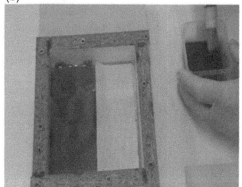 (c) 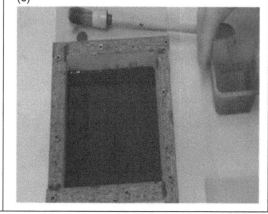

Tips for making and using the model

- Wear gloves (and an apron)
- Spread the layers evenly
- Record/note the curing times
- Involve students in the process of making the model

Supporting learning resources for use when teaching/learning with the model

- Horizontal mattress sutures (https://www. youtube.com/watch?v=HsDZjtK8vWw)
- Vertical mattress suture pattern (https://www. youtube.com/watch?v=e4HM0EEIytM)
- Video of how to make a silicon skin pad (www.wiley.com/go/read/veterinary)

Acknowledgments

The development of the model was funded by the Federal Ministry of Education and Research (Germany).

SimSpay Model

Rikke Langebæk

Department of Veterinary Clinical Science, University of Copenhagen, Copenhagen, Denmark

Ingredients for making the model	Anatomical structure	Where to source
• 1 × disposable instrument tray/ food container. Not too deep	Abdominal cavity	
• 2 × long modelling balloons	Uterus	www.viborg-ballon.dk Model: 30MP
• 2 × short tube balloons	Peritoneal lining	www.viborg-ballon.dk Model: 1LD
• 2 × disposable wash sponge	Infundibulum	
• 1 × red rubber band, 25 cm diam.	Uterine vessels	https://hcemballage.dk/ Model: (5-252-020-1H) 250x2x2
• 2 × ½ red rubber band, 25 cm diam.	Ovarian vessels	
• 2 × brown rubber band, 25 cm diam.	Suspensory ligament and round ligament	https://hcemballage.dk/ Model: (2-200-020-1P) 200 × 2
• 1 × brown rubber band, 25 cm diam.	Ureters	
• 3 × disposable examination glove	Urinary bladder & omentum	
• 1 disposable dish cloth	Abdominal wall	
• Leukoplast Sleek LF (or other sturdy adhesive tape)		https://www.bsnmedical. co.uk/
• Stapler		
• Scissors		

Veterinary Clinical Skills, First Edition. Edited by Emma K. Read, Matt R. Read, and Sarah Baillie.
© 2022 John Wiley & Sons, Inc. Published 2022 by John Wiley & Sons, Inc.
Companion website: www.wiley.com/go/read/veterinary

Steps for Making the Model

1. **Abdominal cavity:** For fixation of abdominal organs make 8 small holes (2–3mm) in the bottom of the instrument tray/food container, 2 larger holes (5–6mm) in the diaphragm end and one large hole (5–6mm) in the pelvis end. Use small sharp scissors for the small holes and a mosquito haemostat for the large holes.	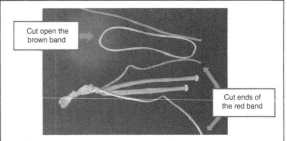 Diaphragm end — Pelvis end
2. **Ovarium and uterus:** The 2 long balloons are tied together with two common knots at 7.5 cm and 3 cm from the closed end. The balloons illustrate the uterine body and horns. Include the red rubber band in the 7.5 cm knot and cut open the loop of this band (Figure 1).	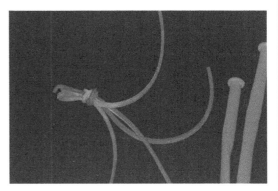 Cut open the brown band Cut ends of the red band **Figure 1**
Tie one of the ends of the red rubber band together with one brown rubber band and ½ red rubber band in a single knot (Figure 2). Cut open the free loop of the brown rubber band (see Figure 1)	**Figure 2**

Cut off the closed end of one short balloon and with a hemostat pull it over the tied together balloons, covering both knots (3 and 7.5 cm knots) plus part of the two strands of the red rubber band. The two red strands should leave the short balloon (peritoneal lining) on each side of the uterus/uterine horns, illustrating the two uterine arteries (Figure 3).

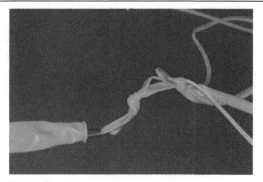

Figure 3

Each end of the long balloon (the tip of the uterine horn) is tied around the combined rubber bands as close to the knot as possible (Figure 4).

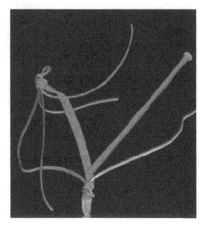

Figure 4

A 5 × 2.5 cm piece of the disposable wash sponge (illustrating the infundibulum) is folded around the balloon and rubber band knots so that one brown rubber band points cranial (the suspensory ligament), while the rest (round ligament (brown), uterine and ovarian vessels (red) points caudal (Figure 5).

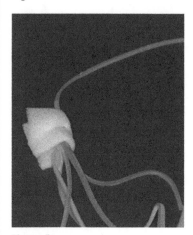

Figure 5

3. **Urinary bladder:**

The fingers of the glove are closed separately with a knot (Figure 6a) and the glove is turned inside-out and stuffed with a disposable wash sponge.

Tie a knot at the sleeve of the glove.

Cut off the closed end of a short balloon (peritoneal lining) and with the hemostat pull the sleeve end of the glove, the knot, and a brown rubber band (urethers) into the balloon.

Cut open the free loop of the rubber band (Figure 6b).

You now have the bladder (Figure 6c).

(a)

(b)

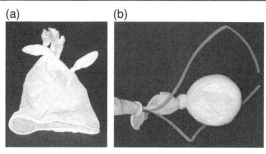

Figure 6a   **Figure 6b**

(c)

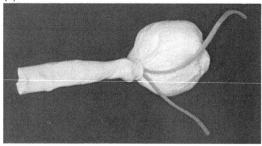

Figure 6c

4. **Placing the organs**

   "Pelvis" end of tray: Put the two "balloon-organs" (bladder and uterus) together, with the bladder "fundus" on top and with a hemostat pull their ends through the large hole in the pelvis end of the tray (Figure 7).

   "Diaphragm" end of tray: With a hemostat pull one glove through each hole, leaving the hand and fingers inside the abdominal cavity, illustrating the omentum (Figure 9 - see next page).

   Bottom of tray: In each side, the cranial brown rubber band (suspensory ligament) is pulled through the bottom hole nearest the diaphragm end, using a hemostat. Leave the rubber band approx. 3 cm long and fix it to the outside with the adhesive tape.

   In each side, the ½ red rubber band (ovarian vessel) is pulled through the middle hole and fixed to the outside with tape. Leave the rubber band approx. 4 cm long.

   The last brown rubber band coming from the infundibulum (round ligament) is pulled through the holes nearer the pelvis end of the tray. Leave the bands rather loose – approx. 10 cm long. Fix to the outside with tape.

   Finally, the two brown rubber bands coming from the bladder (urethers) are pulled through the small holes nearest to the pelvis end and fixed to the outside with tape.

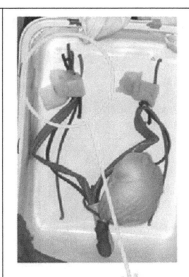

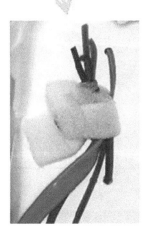

Figure 7

5. **Abdominal wall**

   Staple a disposable kitchen cloth (abdominal fascia) to the edge of the instrument tray, so that it covers the abdominal cavity/tray. Use heavy stationary staples (Figure 8).

   If you want more abdominal wall layers, use additional kitchen cloths or sponge cloths

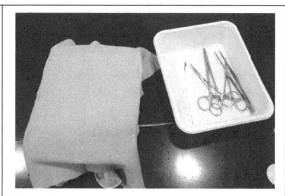

Figure 8

   See Figure 9 for completed model with reproductive tract, bladder and associated structures in situ.

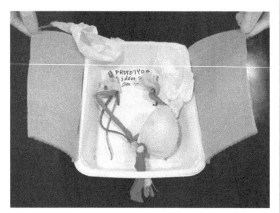

Figure 9

Top Tips for Making and Using the Model

- The model is quite light weight when finished, so it is helpful to strap it to the table with duct tape or construct a stuffed toy animal with a cavity, into which the model can be fixed.
- It is important to let the students build the model themselves, as it helps them obtain an anatomical understanding of the procedure. You can print out an anatomical illustration to go with the materials.
- We suggest using the model prior to students' first elective surgeries/spays. We use it as a test of student competency and to give them more confidence, as they can communicate any doubts or insecurities and receive feedback.

Supporting learning resources for use when teaching/learning with the model

- Video demonstrating the building of the SimSpay http://youtu.be/DGk24utOIfo
- Video performing an ovariohysterectomy on the model http://youtu.be/y0DzB6u9beg

Acknowledgments

The SimSpay was originally master minded by Associate prof. Thomas Eriksen, DVM, PhD, Department of Veterinary Clinical Science, University of Copenhagen.

Reference

Langebæk, R., Toft, N., Eriksen, T. 2015. The SimSpay – student perceptions of a low-cost build-it-yourself model for novice training of surgical skills in canine ovariohysterectomy. *J Vet Med Educ*, 42, 2, 166–171. doi: v10.3138/jvme.1014-105.

Surgical Prep Model

Jean-Yin Tan and Alfredo E. Romero

Faculty of Veterinary Medicine, University of Calgary, Calgary, Alberta, Canada

Ingredients for making the model	
• Camel or brown faux fur fabric to simulate the unclipped hair of the patient ("fur")	Approximately 14×14" (36×36 cm) fabric square. Long fur (pile at least 1″) is preferable, so that it would be dragged into the simulated skin when improper technique is employed. Can be purchased at a fabric store or online (keyword search "long pile fur fabric" or "shaggy fur fabric").
• Brown faux leather fabric to simulate the clipped skin of the patient ("skin")	Approximately 8×8″ (20×20 cm) fabric square. Can be purchased at a fabric store or online (keyword search "faux leather," "pleather," or "synthetic leather").
• Glo Germ	Glo Germ powder and gel (http://www.glogerm.com/mm5/merchant.mvc?Screen=CTGY&Category_Code=PGAOL)
• Blacklight	
• Fabric scissors	Sharp fabric scissors
• Measuring tape	
• 4 sewing fabric pins	
• Needle and strong upholstery thread, heavy-duty sewing machine, or fabric glue	Due to the thickness of the faux fur and leather fabric, a heavy duty sewing or quilting machine and strong upholstery thread should be used.

Veterinary Clinical Skills, First Edition. Edited by Emma K. Read, Matt R. Read, and Sarah Baillie.
© 2022 John Wiley & Sons, Inc. Published 2022 by John Wiley & Sons, Inc.
Companion website: www.wiley.com/go/read/veterinary

Steps for Making the Model

1 The model represents the furry area on a dog that has been previously clipped and must now prepped and/or draped for surgery. The "fur" surrounds the faux leather "skin," which has previously been "clipped." The candidate's job is to perform a surgical prep. To create the model, use fabric scissors to cut an approximately 5×5″ (12×12 cm) rectangular hole in the fur.	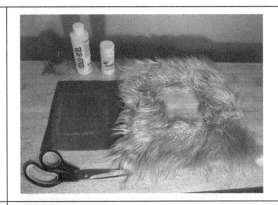
2 Using the sewing fabric pins, attach the simulator skin to the fabric using the outline of the hole as a guide. Attach the 2 fabrics together using a heavy-duty sewing machine, needle, and strong upholstery thread, or fabric glue.	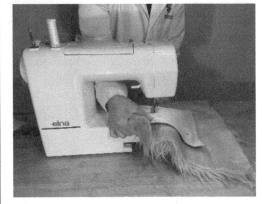 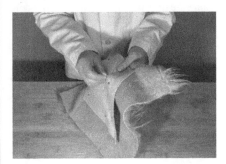 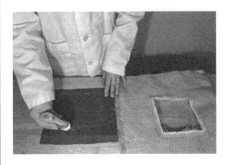

3 Final product after sewing the skin to the fur.	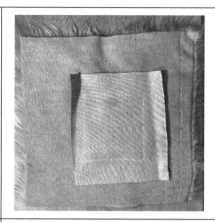
4 Sprinkle Glo Germ powder onto the simulator skin.	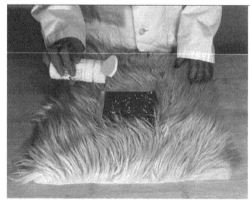
5 Using a gloved hand, smear the Glo Germ gel along the fur surrounding the skin. Ensure some of the hair is dragged onto the simulator skin, which is representing the clipped area that must be surgically prepped.	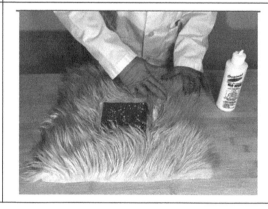

6 After the student has performed the surgical prep, use a black light to examine the simulator skin. Any fluorescence is indicative of contamination. Fluorescence under black light is indicative of contamination (as shown top right corner in the photo).

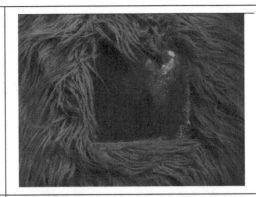

7 The model can also be used for open gloving and draping. If the model is to be reused, wipe the area with a damp towel and repeat Steps 4–5.

The photo shows the model being used in an OSCE station for surgical prep and draping.

If using this model for assessment purposes, it helps to have 1 or 2 extra simulators available to prepare the Glo Germ on the next simulator and to use damp towels to wipe remaining Glo Germ off used simulators.

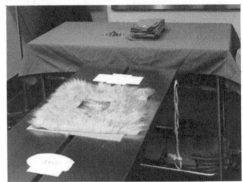

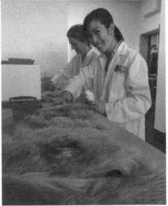

8 Model after surgical draping.

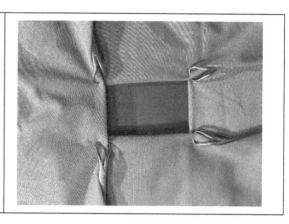

Top Tips for Making and Using the Model

- The fabric is thick and will require a heavy-duty sewing machine and stronger upholstery thread to attach the faux leather.
- Based on trial and error, the combination of Glo Germ powder on the skin and Glo Germ gel on the fur seems to be most effective.

Acknowledgment

The authors would like to acknowledge their colleague Rebecca Archer.

Tea Towel Suturing Model

Alison Catterall

Bristol Veterinary School, University of Bristol, Bristol, United Kingdom

Ingredients for making the model	Where to source the materials
• Household tea towel × 1 (the type that has a checked lines pattern)	Available from most homeware shops and supermarkets
• Gauze swab × 1 (10 cm × 10 cm)	Used for wound dressing
• Pair of scissors	
• Clip board × 1	Available from most stationers
• Bulldog clips × 3	Available from most stationers

Steps for Making the Model

1 Cut the tea towel in half – each half (approximately 40 cm × 50 cm) will make a suturing model.	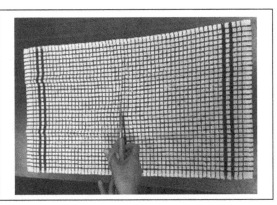

Veterinary Clinical Skills, First Edition. Edited by Emma K. Read, Matt R. Read, and Sarah Baillie.
© 2022 John Wiley & Sons, Inc. Published 2022 by John Wiley & Sons, Inc.
Companion website: www.wiley.com/go/read/veterinary

2 Place a gauze swab in the center of the tea towel.	
3 Fold the outer edges of the tea towel inwards to the edge of the gauze swab, but do not cover the swab.	
4 Fold the outer edges (again) into the middle and over the gauze swab (where the folded edges will meet). The gauze swab is now hidden under the edges of the tea towel.	
5 To make the incision (which is approximately 10 cm in length), staple the edges of the tea towel together. Ensure the lines of the tea towel match up exactly across the incision (as the lines are used for guidance when suturing).	

6 Place three staples (one behind the other) at either end of the "incision."

   Do not staple the gauze swab (the staples will sit on top of the pad).

   The white lines show the position of staples.

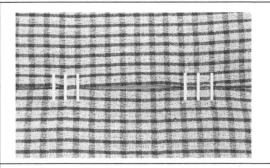

7 Place the tea towel on the clip board using the board's clip to anchor it at one end and two bulldog clips to anchor it at the other end.

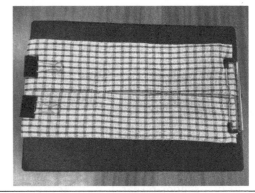

Tips for making and using the model

An extra bulldog clip, fixed to a tabletop, can be used to stop the board moving around while it is in use.

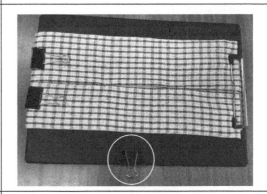

Dying the tea towel a darker color helps to see the sutures when using white suture material, e.g. monofilament nylon on a reel (which may be used in the clinical skills laboratory as it is cheaper than other suture materials).

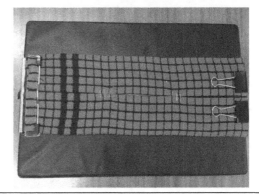

Ensuring the lines of the tea towel are aligned across the wound will ensure the sutures are being positioned correctly to close the wound

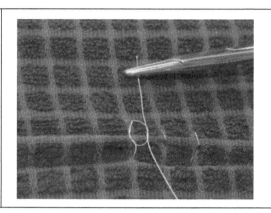

Supporting learning resources for use when teaching/learning with the model

- Suturing instruction booklet: www.bristol. ac.uk/vet-school/research/comparative-clinical/veterinary-education/clinical-skills-booklets/sutures/

Paper about the model

Baillie, S., Christopher, R., Catterall, A., et al. 2019. Comparison of a silicon skin pad and a tea towel for learning a simple interrupted suture. *J Vet Med Educ*. Advance online. doi: https://doi.org/10.3138/jvme.2018-0001.

Index

Veterinary Clinical Skills, First Edition. Edited by Emma K. Read, Matt R. Read, and Sarah Baillie.
© 2022 John Wiley & Sons, Inc. Published 2022 by John Wiley & Sons, Inc.
Companion website: www.wiley.com/go/read/veterinary